Sub

A quest for the .

This is the story of one man's quest to achieve the
improbable goal of running a sub three-hour marathon
while holding down a big international business career
and bringing up a small family. Many have tried, few
have succeeded. Fewer still have succeeded many
times.

.

A road is for running

no matter how far or fast you run it.

Andy Bass

With special thanks to my wife, friends, family, colleagues, contributors, collaborators, and fellow runners known and unknown, who have inspired, supported, endured, and celebrated this improbable quest over several decades.

First published in Great Britain 2023
This paperback edition published 2023

Copyright © Andy Bass 2023

ISBN Paperback: 978-1-3999-5477-8

CONTENTS

Sub-3

A quest for the improbable

Sub-3

A quest for the improbable

According to Google about 1.1 million people per year complete a marathon which is just 0.01 percent of the world's population. According to marastats.com less than 4% of all marathon runners ever manage to break three hours for this distance.

This book is dedicated to all those amateur athletes from all walks of sporting life who have ever attempted, or are thinking of attempting, a Sub-3 marathon.

This is one man's quest for that legendary status and the addiction to do it again and again. From what began as a laddish challenge at the age of twenty-nine, and an uncertified run at The London Marathon in 1990, to over twenty-five years of running over one hundred marathons of all types in all sorts of terrain and all around the world.

This is an anecdotal guide to what it takes, and how long it may take, if you are not a serious runner but run to keep fit to play other sports and like a drink or two throughout the week.

It is a book about building your sport around your life rather than your life around your sport. It is not a guide to help you with nutrition and fitness and tactics, and a training plan. It's simply a catalogue of selected events across twenty-five years of memories, forfeits, bets, and consequences for failing the task. It's not about taking yourself seriously, but it is about chasing a serious goal.

You will know many people who have run a marathon, but you will know few people who have gone Sub-3, and even fewer who have done it multiple times that are not otherwise part of a serious athletics club.

I have friends who have completed numerous Ironman races, and even qualified for the Ironman Kona World Championships but have not cracked a Sub-3 marathon. I have other friends who are seriously fit from football, rugby, rowing, and other high-energy sports that have tried but failed to hit the Sub-3 mark.

For those of you who think you must become a serious club athlete to make a Sub-3 then think again, for those of you who think you have to give up drink and calories for six months or a year then think again.

I have never weighed less than seventy-three kilos and have typically run at three or four kilos heavier than that. I look more like Gazza than I do Steve Cram.

The night before a run would typically involve a Guinness, or two. I have a terrible gag reflex so serious nutrition for me is a big no-no, and just the smell of bananas has me reaching for the big white telephone.

My early years were spent playing amateur football two or three times a week with the usual Tuesday and Thursday night training. At the age of twenty-nine I switched to playing rugby, at forty-three I switched to triathlon.

Marathons were simply a side hobby to my main sport at the time. I had a high-profile business career managing a large corporation, regularly travelling all around the world, a wife, two kids, a couple of dogs and a Volvo. So, nothing special to see here just someone living a "normal" business and sporting life who added marathon running to his annual schedule of things to do and the quest to go Sub-3 as part of that challenge.

I hope you find some things that resonate with your own quest to have either failed or succeeded this challenge or if you are still in pursuit of it. I hope you will see that no two journeys will ever be the same and, despite the hundreds of books available on how to run a marathon, and all the different sorts of training guides and race plans, I can honestly say I never read one.

You must simply find your own way, your own style and work with your own unique circumstances. You can do this, no matter what age you start trying.

You may need to adapt your life around it but the day you do it will be a special one and you will be part of that exclusive Sub-3 club.

A road is for running no matter how far or fast you run it.

Don't give up.

1. London Marathon 1990

The Start of Something!

In 1990, at the age of twenty-nine, I ran my first marathon. A friend asked, "What's your target time?" "Sub-3" I said without hesitation. His eyebrows raised.

"Have you run a marathon before" he said. "Nope" I replied. "What sort of training have you done?" he asked. "Well, I do rugby training twice a week, play every Saturday and run the river loop from Hammersmith to Barnes three times a week in just over thirty minutes" I replied confidently.

"Like how much over 30 minutes?" he pressed. "Say 32-33 minutes give or take" I said. "So, you just have to do six or seven river loops at that same pace give or take?" he countered "Er yeah, is it that many loops?" I replied, trying to do the math.

"Hmmm" he said, "and the race is a week on Sunday?" "Yep, all ready to go" I replied. "Ok he said, and are we having any side bets on this?" "Well, it's a done deal", I said, "Real men finish in under three hours, and everyone else finishes after that" I blurted out. "OK, so you are saying that only real men finish in under three hours and presumably all women and those that aren't real men finish after three hours?"

I could feel some sort of trap emerging. "Well yeah, except for the professional women, and the really fast club women runner types" I said trying to recover my earlier claim. "So, if you don't go under three hours that effectively means you are not a real man?" he continued. "Well yes, I guess it does now you put it like that", I replied. "So, let's set the bet at if you don't go under three hours then you will wear a dress next Friday night at The Rutland?" he offered, and the trap was set. "OK done", I confidently replied as this wasn't going to happen. I would be wearing a Sub-3 finisher shirt down the pub on Friday, and they would be buying my drinks all night.

Getting a slot in the London Marathon via the ballot is particularly hard. I have never managed to get one despite more than twenty years of trying. I entered the first ever London Marathon in 1981, the first year it was established. Me and a few friends thought it would be a good idea and we applied. This is years before mobile phones, computers, or any form of modern-day technology. Places were limited then as they are now.

The process was to request an entry form which we received by post. The entry had to be posted back but not before a specific date and time. The entry slot would be first come first served based on the postmark date and time of the submitted entry after midnight on a specific date. I remember going to Northampton town centre Post Office just before midnight and posting all three applications dead on midnight. That should do it.

A few days later we all received rejection letters and I seem to remember that the race sold out by 2am postmarked letters the following day. Although we had posted the letters through the main post office letter box at midnight, the chances are they weren't processed until a few hours after or even the following morning.

That was the start of over twenty years of entering the ballot and never getting accepted. The conditions and requirements changed over time, but the result was always the same. Every year I paid for the entry fee and ticked the box saying they could keep it for charity if I didn't get in, and every year, I got one of those consolation training tops which signified to the world that you hadn't received a ballot place.

Getting an official entry would mean applying for a charity place or via some sort of qualification process. I'm not exactly sure when the Good for Age entry came into play, but essentially you had to prove a Sub-3 marathon if you were, say under forty years of age and a Sub-3:15 marathon if you were, say over forty.

Qualification times had to be from a recognised marathon. So how come I am running London in 1990? Well officially, I'm not. Me and a close friend (aka Sauce) decided to turn up and run it anyway. Jump the barrier and join in.

I'm not condoning that behaviour , I'm not proud of it, but at the end of the day I am simply running from Blackheath to Westminster on the same day as the London Marathon and the only difference is those around me have a number and a timing chip and I don't.

The plan was to meet at Sauce's place in Walton-On-Thames the night before, have a pasta dinner, get an early night, and another friend (aka Wildman) would drive us to Blackheath the morning after that and we would work it out from there.

A slight problem arose a few days before the race. I had recently become single from a long-term girlfriend and had started a new job. I was particularly attracted to someone who was working with our company for an external agency. Following an after-work event and to my pleasant surprise, we ended up agreeing to meet for a drink that Saturday, the night before the race.

As much as I respect sporting records and performance, a Sub-3 challenge is not top of mind at this stage, and running a marathon was neither here nor there faced with the alternative of a night out with her. Sauce had left a key on a string inside the letter box of his flat in case I might make it. Despite my late-night party state, and after a two-hour drive, I arrived at his place around 2am, let myself in and crashed out on his sofa in the front room.

At 6am I was woken up by Sauce who was ecstatic I had made it and the race was on. A while later, he was sitting in the kitchen eating plain pasta from a saucepan which he had just boiled and was asking me if I wanted some. I had no idea why anyone would want to eat that at any time of the day let alone for breakfast. He had read somewhere that eating pasta was a key marathon running requirement.

On the way to Blackheath in the car he offered me a variety of energy tablets, salt tablets and whatever else he had read up on. I simply wanted water and an open window to puke out of.

At Blackheath the roads were all being closed, and Wildman got us as close as he could to the Blackheath Common before we bailed out and joined the rest of the runners walking to the start. Dressed in old T-shirts and track suit bottoms to dump at the start, and plastic bin liners to wear over us to stay warm and disguise the fact we had no numbers, we jumped a couple of barriers and mingled in with the registered runners.

The plan was to meet at Big Ben after the race and meet Wildman at a designated pub away from Westminster. With a minute to go before the start, old T-Shirts, track suits and bin liners were being discarded around us before we set off into the chaos of the official runners and us simply running on public roads albeit on the marathon course.

You may get to run the course from Blackheath to Westminster Bridge (now The Mall) but you won't cross the finish line without a number or a tag. Just when you are approaching the finish and waving to the adoring crowds you must run the gauntlet of security. This is not a group of bouncers in bow ties and knuckle dusters, but a long line of track-suited fast runner types focussed on anyone without a number. They pick you off as quickly as the creatures in the film A Quiet Place.

I did this a few times before I earned a Good for Age slot but never once beat that line of security near the finish. They are very good at what they do so take it from me, don't bother. To be honest, there aren't a huge number of unofficial runners, a dozen or more at most so to all those claiming it's theft of someone else's water on the course then please spare me the judgement. I already paid for it via the entry fee and there will be ten times as many DNF's and DNS's than there will be idiots like me running without a number.

I clearly don't have an official time from then, but I was pulled off the course around three hours and twenty-two minutes with another five-hundred yards to go so a forfeit for failure was now required based on the "real man" problem since created.

I sat by Big Ben freezing to death waiting over an hour or two for Sauce to arrive. A couple, waiting for their son to run past, kindly lent me a jacket to keep warm.

This was indeed the start of something.

I sat reflecting on the pending time penalty and the consequences of not going Sub-3 but more so on how I had held the pace to half-way and how the time had slipped away fast during the second half. Was this a mental issue, a physical issue, or both? One thing was certain, I had caught the bug and I would be back.

That following Friday my close friend Amanda selected an appropriate dress for me to wear for the evening with a variety of accessories, a pair of her old tights and some make-up.

I made it through the night relatively unscathed despite a late-night scuffle with a mate who kept pinching my arse, but all in all the start of something began with a disrespectful claim that running a Sub-3 marathon is a slam dunk for any self-respecting sportsman.

In my case it was the claim for every marathon thereafter for years to come and the forfeits and complexity of penalties kept coming.

Whereas the 1990 London Marathon was the start of something, the 2017 London Marathon, over twenty-five years later, would turn out to be the end of something.

The years between would be a long string of Sub-3 attempts and forfeits and a sports challenge companion for life.

2. New York Marathon 1990
Imperfect Preparation

Following the unofficial running of the London Marathon six months earlier, my running partner in crime (Sauce) and the getaway driver (Wildman) decided to sign up for the New York Marathon via a travel firm type package as that seemed to be the only way to get an official entry.

Usual rules would apply. No special training was allowed outside of standard football and rugby, no abstinence from normal drinking in the run up to and including the night before the race, Sub-3 finish or some sort of forfeit.

We arrived on the Friday for the race on Sunday and struggled our way through the various complexities of registering. To our dismay, getting to the start on time was early, very early. Buses to the start line across the Verrazano bridge were running from 5am and stopping at 6am.

Runners would be held at the start area hours before the start time in the freezing cold. But hey, we're in New York, we're all young, free and single and we are flying back a day after the race so let's enjoy it.

The agreement was to have one or two beers on Saturday night and get to bed early for the race on Sunday, so we left the hotel to find a bar. This probably went on for a beer too many, but as we were walking back to the hotel around 10pm, we passed a bar with bouncers outside on the sidewalk.

We thought, why not one last nightcap but luckily the bouncers said it was a private party. We thanked them and were about to move on when they asked why we were in New York City. We mentioned the pending marathon and after a short conversation they were so impressed they let us in. Well, it's just one more and back to the hotel right! I went to the bar to get a final round and asked for the bill only to find out it was a free bar! I know what you're thinking. A free bar!

After a few more rounds, we staggered back to the hotel around 2am and to this day I have no idea who managed to get us up at 4am for breakfast and onto the buses but they did. We slept on the bus and later on a grass bank at the start area as the New York Marathon sun was rising and waking up the race.

We passed the time watching people stretching out and going through their final pre-race preparations. We marvelled at the makeshift men's urinals arrangement which was an open-air section of downhill rain guttering about three hundred yards long where it seemed safer to pee as far upstream as possible than risk a downstream soaking. We locked a few people in the Portaloo's for the fun of it and waited to see who would let them out before we ambled off to the start-line.

Sub-3 anyone? No chance, not even if we had gone to bed sober at 6pm. Despite our condition I finished in 3:16 with the other two in 3:36 and 4:32. Going Sub-3 was now two down and zero.

3.   London Marathon 1991
Failure and forfeit

For the London Marathon 1991, the forfeit for not going Sub-3 was a pint of Carling Premier for every five minutes over three hours, plus a chaser of their choosing and a Prawn Fahl at the Spice of Night on the south side of Hammersmith Bridge. The forfeit would be rounded up not down, mates can be quite creative.

On race day, Wildman duly drove me early morning from the West side of London over to Blackheath, manoeuvring in an out of the road closures and dropping me off about an hour or so before the start.

Dodging security to get inside the red start area was relatively straight forward. Getting unchallenged into a starting pen was a little more difficult but once the masses were massing it was relatively straight forward to run alongside everyone and have a plan to get out before the finish where the bouncers would be waiting.

A typical 'too fast' start to get me to halfway at around the 1:30 mark would be followed by the dawning reality of a second half meltdown and my estimated finish time, having been taken off by the bouncers at the finish, was 3:28.

Wildman had offered to pick me up in Green Park after the race and give me a 'backer' home to Hammersmith, five miles away, on his push-bike. This generous offer lasted all of two minutes as my backside was on fire from dangling off the seat of the bike and the decision was taken to reverse roles and that I would cycle him back instead. Perhaps a quick swim in the Thames afterwards and we could have invented a new sport called triathlon!

A 3:28 finish meant this would be rounded up to 3:30 under the rounding-up rule and it would therefore mean a penalty of six pints of Carling Premier and six chasers of their choosing.

Having downed the first pint, they congregated at the bar to discuss the chaser. I was expecting gin or whisky or some spirit I simply can't handle. They came up with another pint of Carling Premier as the Chaser, and needless to say, I slept on the floor of the curry house having collapsed after three or four pints and follow up chasers and a couple of mouthfuls of a Prawn Fahl, which looked more like tar than a curry house dish.

Maybe this was 'Men Behaving Badly' and maybe this is not a typical running club (none of them were runners) but maybe looking back this implanted the enormity of a Sub-3 on all of us Friday-night piss-up mortals.

A runner's respect was breaking out amongst rugby, football, and cricket types alike. Over the years most of them would attempt a marathon at some point in their life and to this day I am not aware of any of them coming close to four hours let alone going Sub-3.

4.   London Marathon 1993

A Charity Place

Getting into The London Marathon on the ballot is next to impossible. I don't know a single person, except Mystic Chris (see Chapter 8), who tried that got in. Of the 35,000 runners, only 1,000 or so are Good for Age or Elite qualify so the rest must be celebrity slots and charity places. To run for a charity, you need to raise £2-3,000 so that the charity can recover the £600-£700 it has had to pay for the entry in the first place. You can tap your friends and family up for sponsorship for one year, or maybe two before it starts to get a bit tiresome for them and for you.

Up until a few years ago there was a window of opportunity to apply for the race over a few days or so and the ballot would lock out at a certain level of entries, say 50,000, who knows. Then it changed to a much longer period to enter and no limit of entries. According to a google search, a record number of 457,861 people entered the ballot for the 2020 London Marathon. The ballot is completely random and around 17,000 get a ballot place which is just 3.71%.

In each case you are asked if you want to donate your entry fee to charity if you are unsuccessful in gaining an entry. I suspect most people tick the "Yes" box thinking if you tick "No" you might stand less of a chance at getting a place. The entry fee is now £49 so if 50% of entrants tick Yes to donate then that amounts to £10M from runners who won't be running. If they charge charities £600 or more for charity places and there are 20,000 of those then that's another £12M earned so that's a decent turnover for a charity that made £35M turnover in 2021.

In the years I ran for charity I think I simply made up the difference with £500-£600 of my own money as I only have so many friends and family and time to make cakes for a cake stall to cover it. Up to the 1990's when the ballot entry was closed after a few days, around 30% of those applying made the ballot to run.

Today it is probably less than 4% so it's no longer worth trying in my opinion. My advice is to find another race like Dublin or another major city marathon and work on a Good for Age slot for London although I understand they are making that harder too.

I tried to find my finish time for 1993 but there aren't any websites going back that far. I was about to give up when I found a book on Amazon called The London Marathon – 1993. How bizarre. A one-hundred-and-twenty-page full colour picture book with hundreds of images of the race plus about fifty pages of individual finisher times covering 25.000 finishers.

Optimistically, I started at 3:15 and worked my way down from there and I was pleasantly surprised to find myself at 3:19:53 so all in all not a bad time but not even close to the real goal. If nothing else I now have a whole book to read that covers just that one race.

5.   The Wilderness Years 1993-2002

Frank Bruno

There were a lot of life and sport changes for me going on throughout the 1990's and to the millennium. A change of job, a move to London, a new sport from football to rugby, work promotions, marriage, kids, and emigrating to California in late 1997 where we lived for three years before returning to London at the end of 2000.

Routine sport and fitness carried on in the background with the focus on playing rugby (back to football in the USA) and with three of four five mile runs each week to keep fit to play well. Being in my thirties and moving to forty by the end of the decade was beginning to show up in my main sports performance though remarkably, I had never suffered major injury save for a broken collar bone, smashed up eye and concussion here and there. I don't remember a week where I didn't get to run after work most nights in between rugby training and playing at the weekend.

I don't know how many times I ran the London marathon unofficially throughout the 90's, maybe four, or five but I never kept a record; all I know is that I always ran around a 3:30 race and took myself off the course somewhere near Big Ben so that I didn't have to run the gauntlet of the bouncers closer to the finish.

We moved to California to live for a few years where I teamed up with a Michelin Star French Chef, who was the husband of my wife's best friend, and together we ran several US marathons in LA, San Diego, and Long Beach.

He also had the Sub-3 bug, and his times were a good ten to fifteen minutes quicker than mine but suffice to say, each race for both parties ended in disappointment. Times of 3:22, 3:36 and even a shocking 3:49 felt like it was becoming clear to me in my late thirties that the Sub-3 dream was well and truly over, and maybe I should give up trying and do something else.

Returning to London from California, I ran my last uncertified London Marathon in 2002. I managed to hop the start barrier at the Blue Start and mix in with the other runners in the pen about 100 yards from the start line. I was covered in a black bin liner, wearing a black beanie, and keeping in the middle of the start group away from the roving eyes of the start marshals who were scanning for imposters like me.

There was still fifteen minutes to the start of the race and so far, so good, keeping the low profile looked like I would be fine. Other runners were coming into the pen making it more congested and harder to be detected. With about five minutes to go I heard this familiar loud guffawing laugh from someone standing right behind me.

I chose not to turn round as I am not wanting attention drawn to myself. Soon there is another loud familiar laugh and I heard someone else right behind me say "Have a good one Frank".

The next thing I know, Frank Bruno is literally standing right next to me. I tried to ignore him as the marshals were now realising who he was and taking some interest, in him, not me. In hindsight maybe he was great cover, as I am now simply hiding in plain sight.

To my surprise, he asked me where the Start Line was, and I pointed to a big banner about 100 yards ahead of us which said START in huge letters. He laughed and then looked down at me in my black bin liner and black beanie and boomed in his loud voice "You look like you're about to rob a bank". How we laughed, well he did, loudly again.

In 1986 I had stayed up late while at University to listen to the Bruno V Witherspoon fight on the radio from the USA and shouted "Go on Frank" at the radio throughout the whole contest. Only Boxing and Rowing come above running in terms of sheer physical exhaustion and I fell in love with boxing as a teenager watching the Ali versus Frazier fights. I was devastated the following morning following Frank's defeat in the 11th round of fifteen in those days, and his usual humble and dignified nature in defeat.

I wrote him a letter simply addressed to Frank Bruno, Royal Oak Gym, Canning Town, London as a show of support and that he shouldn't give up but keep going. I've no idea if he got it but to be standing next to a real sporting hero before the start of the marathon was very special. Frank finished in 4:47:16 carrying over 100kg of weight across that 26.2-mile course.

I can honestly say no-one carrying that kind of weight will ever go Sub-3 in a marathon, nor could they, nor should they. Eliud Kipchoge weighs in at 52kg so he would have to carry himself on his back for a comparative time against Frank.

Any runner would certainly go Sub-3 in the ring with Frank, it being just a question of when he would land a punch in the first round. In a way Frank had a different Sub-3 achievement vs us mortals.

I ran my typical 3:25 or 3:30 or whatever it was having paced a Sub-3 to halfway and as usual and as always had blown up and slipped drastically in the second half of the race. I probably started the walk and run routine from fifteen, or sixteen-miles in.

The early 2000's were starting as the late 90's had finished, with a typical and predictable attempt and failure. Having crossed the forty years old line a couple of years earlier then surely, for me at least, the Sub-3 dream was dead and buried.

6.   London Marathon 2003

Wild Horses

In January 2003 a bunch of us, including Rhino Guy (more later), decided to attempt the original mud run called Tough Guy on Mr Mouse farm in Wolverhampton, set on a farm for rescued animals and run by Mr Mouse who resembled Windsor Davies from 'It Ain't Arf hot mum'.

A few thousand eccentric runners ran the ultimate obstacle course in the deep freeze of winter, through underwater tunnels, fires, electric shock tunnels, high plunges into lakes with frogmen for safety, up and down anthill runs, with nothing more than a cup of Bovril and pneumonia at the end of it. A real classic and a January event scheduled for us for three of four years in a row.

Runners were corralled into groups; the 'Front Squad' who were positioned at the front and at the base of the start hill, 'Tough Guy' set half-way further back up the hill and a variety of other start groups like 'Wobble Muckers' and 'Dip Shits' starting even further back at the top of the start hill and beyond.

Runners were required to sign a no-fault-form or waiver called a "death warrant" before the start that would absolve the organisers of any liability. Most ran in thermals and gloves, some in nothing more than a thong, others in wedding dresses and some carrying various large objects and the like. A crazy pantomime of characters half drowning, half shivering, half getting electrocuted or cut by broken ice and smoked to death through burning hay bales along the way.

In the car on the way back to London, someone commented that this was indeed the hardest race in the world, and we were all indeed hard and tough guys, plus of course the tough women who were also in it with us.

After a short-lived consensus of this indeed being the hardest and toughest race in the world, someone in the back said, "No I think there's something else which is harder called Steelman or Bronzeman or something like that".

My ears pricked up and looking in the mirror behind me I asked what it was. "I'm not totally sure" came the reply "but it's a long swim, a long bike, and a long run after that, like a marathon so much longer than what we ran today plus a long swim and a bike into the bargain".

And so, I became aware of Ironman for the first time, in the car, caked in mud, driving back from Tough Guy realising there might be something out there tougher than Tough Guy. Rhino Guy also seemed animated by this discussion. This was well before smart phones so no Googling it there and then or anything, just a note to self to do some research.

Within a few days Rhino Guy had discovered this whole new world of Ironman, and what were then only a handful of races listed around the world but with nothing close to home in the UK.

He had found a chance to race Ironman Switzerland that July and that maybe we should sign up for it. He explained the distances and other than running a marathon I had never swam that far before and I didn't own a bike.

That said, each discipline looked doable but maybe not all three at once back-to-back after each other. I was doubtful. Running a marathon was hard enough let alone doing one after all that other stuff. I said no, it's beyond me, but Rhino Guy insisted, and he duly signed up.

To get out of the situation I agreed to sign up if I did well in the London Marathon 2003 which was coming up in a few weeks. I ran a dismal 3:32 and felt pretty much exhausted all the way round and was clearly getting slower with age not faster. Happily, Ironman Switzerland had announced all slots were taken a week or two before London so I couldn't enter anyway. Rhino Guy would have to go solo.

A few weeks later, an e-mail arrived from Rhino Guy saying unbelievably good news, Ironman Switzerland have released an additional 200 slots on a first come first serve basis. Shit. But still having no bike this made little difference to me, so thanks again but no thanks again.

A month later, I was driving into work and stuck in traffic when Wild Horses came on the radio. Something had been bugging me of late, not sure what it was, but the thought of attempting Ironman Switzerland in just eight weeks' time floated into my mind as I was singing to myself in the car. I arrived at work, cancelled my first meetings, and started digging around to see if there were still slots and how to enter.

By lunchtime the event fees were paid, the flight and hotel were booked, and things were locked and loaded. I knew I could run a marathon, albeit it slowly. Time to come up with a training plan!

1. Buy a Bike
2. Cycle London to Brighton and back (180K)
3. Swim 180 lengths of the local pool (3.8K)
4. Enter a Half Ironman as a practise run
5. All set for Switzerland.

It soon became apparent how much kit and preparation you need to do an Ironman. A couple of Rhino Guy's new-found triathlon buddies were doing the race and had done them before, so I quickly latched on to them for hints and tips and what to do, and what not to do.

The day before the race they spent ages in the Expo village buying all sorts of expensive accessories for their bikes and comparing different types of gels and energy bars and wetsuits and goggles and things. One of them bought a carbon water bottle holder which cost about a quarter of the price of my whole bike.

Later they insisted on a practice swim in Lake Zurich, so I eagerly grabbed my 2nd hand wetsuit a work colleague in the USA had given me for surfing. At this point my amateur cover was blown. "What's that?" one of them quipped. "My wetsuit?" I explained with the source of my suit. "Well, it's pretty much useless, you need a wet suit for buoyancy, not to keep you warm, mate!" the other said as he pulled on his shiny full rubber, light-weight suit. "And on top of that the lake is going to be warm so you will burn up in that thing" came the added insight. Ah, schoolboy error No.1, coupled with the fact I could only swim breaststroke, was a wetsuit that would slow me down and heat me up, it was going to be a long day.

I don't know how we did it, but we did. Rhino Guy finished well ahead of me, but I was pleased with my 13:17 finish (that's thirteen hours plus in case you are wondering). I had managed to breaststroke the swim in the wrong type of wetsuit and my trusty new Trek 500 that had cost me about £500 had done me proud.

The Ironman bug had bitten, and with it came the turning point on caring about marathon times. Training was now all based around swimming, biking, and running, not just running. Ironman races, for slow people like me, go on for 11 hours at best and 15 hours at worst, whereas a Sub-3 marathon is what it says on the tin.

The quest for a Sub-10 Ironman is for another time and another book but we soon established certain rules to determine a 'real man' Ironman time from just a standard Ironman time. One rule created was it must include a Sub-4 marathon to make sure the cyclists and the swimmer types didn't simply 'half walk' the run. Of the fifteen Ironman's I have completed only two met that rule, despite running being my strongest discipline on paper.

So, after thirteen years of running to supplement other sports, the focus was changing to the whole new world of Ironman triathlon. Marathons would still be part of that schedule but now marathons were simply training for Ironman.

Marathon times for now were no longer a focus. It seemed clear at the time that running a Sub-3 was never going to happen so why keep chasing it?

Ironman brough a whole new world of friends and venues and gadgets and equipment to buy. Marathons were the past not the future.

7. VO2 Max, Carbs, The Red Zone
Going Nerd

In 2003 my mid-life crisis started to take shape in the form of an Ironman tattoo and travelling the world doing Ironman races. By 2004 it was time to get more serious and immerse myself in the sport. I became all scientific, and with this newfound love I had the medal, the finisher T-shirt, and the tattoo to prove it. I started subscribing to the main triathlon magazine of the time, 220 Triathlon.

It would drop through the door once a month and I would scan through it for tips and gadgets and upcoming events. I would always buy it at the airport so that other passengers could see I was a serious athlete and I studiously flicked through it feeling cool and self-important. It was probably going a bit too far to roll my trouser leg up so that people could see my new Ironman tattoo, but you get the picture.

I was in my early forties, so this was probably part of that mid-life crisis thing without having to buy a new motorbike, which on reflection would have been a lot cheaper. I was so cool that I assumed 220 Triathlon meant going Sub-2:20 for an Olympic Triathlon or something, which didn't seem that fast to me and anyway who does those short distance races anyway?

It was a few months later when I was taken down a peg or two after hearing from others that it was to do with VO2 Max. Of course, I nodded along, having no idea what they were talking about, but the term "VO2 Max" sounded much cooler than a Sub 2:20 Olympic distance triathlon. I mean we all know why GQ is called GQ right? Right?

Having sussed out that VO2 Max was something to do with your age and your heart rate then a whole new world was opening up. Another thing to explore, more gadgets to buy, maybe this is the secret to a Sub-3 marathon. I went down to Waterstones and started flicking through the sections on fitness, training, and well-being. There were plenty of glossy, general texts and books but nothing 'meaty'.

I needed something more in depth, something more intellectual maybe, something well, nerdy, I guess. After a further search there was one book with just the one copy hidden amongst the other best-sellers. No fluff, no fancy pictures, no clever intriguing title to draw you in, just page after page after page of graphs, charts, tables and old black and white pictures of famous cyclists and runners from back in the 60's and 70's.

'Training Lactate Pulse-Rate' by Peter G.J.M Janssen. One hundred and eighty pages of what looked more like a PHD thesis than a book, with sections like "Increase of exertion PR after recent bronchitis in a marathon runner" or "The Oxygen transportation capacity of the blood" or "Extensive example of a field test and training advice for a marathon runner" and even "Intensity Table for runners in meters per second".

This was it. Pure gold. Gathering dust on the shelves at Waterstones and only one copy left, and it was all mine.

How come no-one had found this book before? Maybe they had? Maybe it had sold out and was a best seller. The person on the till struggled for a while to find it on the system so for a short moment I thought I might be deprived of my new treasure. Then, it was in the bag, and I was off back home to work my way through the charts and graphs and make some sense of it of it all.

There was a lot of detail on pulse rate and anaerobic thresholds as well as lactate levels and blood levels and comparisons between cyclists, runners, and sprinters. There was too much to take in and I skipped chapters on "Conconi's Test" and "Determination of the deflection point". I skipped to the most important chapter "The Concept of VO2 Max". I soon discovered it was to do with your maximum heart rate and the point at which you move into the 'red zone' where you will eventually 'bonk' or have a heart attack if you try and hold that level for above say forty minutes or so.

To work out your VO2 Max you simply had to deduct your age from 220 and that was it, as simple as that. So being forty or so my max heart rate should only be 180 during running, rowing, or racing for a very short space of time or face death. If only I had a heart rate monitor that would really help.

There were also guides on your optimal training heart rate range so for me it was about 125-150, again great, if only I had a heart monitor. Now what? What am I supposed to do with that? Lactate! Yep, I've heard of that. Not good I understand. Anaerobic Threshold? That sounded good and plenty of graphs to go with it. Then on Page 115 it all started to click.

Here was a graph of the heart rate of a "failed marathon runner" from the Eindhoven Marathon. The "deflection point" for this person was 165 beats/minute and a Vo2 Max of 180. The graph shows the runner going above 165 almost from the start of the race, climbing to 170 beats/minute by 10K and touching 180 beats by 20K.

The time to 20K was 1:23;27 so halfway would have been about 1:27 (sounding familiar). From 20K the heart rate starts to drop dramatically to 130 beats/minute then back up to 160, back down to 130, back up to 160 and so on. Clearly the runner is now running some and walking some (this is sounding very familiar).

The book says "From the start to the 25th Kilometre, pulse rate is over 165 so the runner can perform about 1 hour and 50 minutes over his deflection point. Then he cannot keep up his pace any longer. Running speed goes down rapidly so does his PR. The first 20K split is covered in 1:23:27 and the second in 1:54:52. Total marathon time is 3:27:28."

And then it all clicked into place. Every marathon I have run for the past fifteen years or so has followed that exact graph. Finally, the science behind a failed Sub-3.

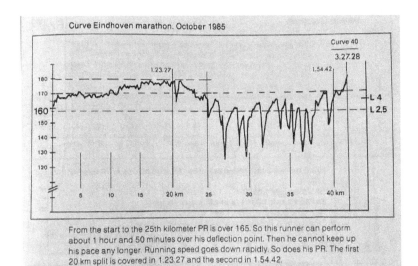

Curve Eindhoven marathon. October 1985

From the start to the 25th kilometer PR is over 165. So this runner can perform about 1 hour and 50 minutes over his deflection point. Then he cannot keep up his pace any longer. Running speed goes down rapidly. So does his PR. The first 20 km split is covered in 1.23.27 and the second in 1.54.42. Total time marathon: 3 h. 27 min. 28 sec.

So, what now? Well according to the book, the same runner was tracked six months later running a different marathon, as below.

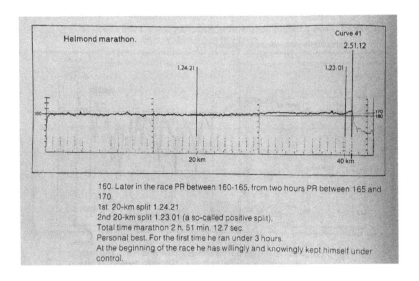

Helmond marathon.

160. Later in the race PR between 160-165, from two hours PR between 165 and 170.
1st 20-km split 1.24.21
2nd 20-km split 1.23.01 (a so-called positive split).
Total time marathon 2 h. 51 min. 12.7 sec.
Personal best. For the first time he ran under 3 hours.
At the beginning of the race he has willingly and knowingly kept himself under control.

All he had to do was keep his pulse rate down below 160 for the entire race and bingo, no going into The Red Zone, a nice smooth run, and a perfect Sub-3 marathon.

So that's it, you don't need to read the rest of the book simply buy yourself a heart monitor, keep a steady pace at or below your deflection point, wave to the crowd and cross the line well inside the dream time. I bought myself a Polar watch. Remember those? They were big before Garmin and Strava and I still have one or two at the bottom of a man drawer somewhere. I set it up to beep at the right mile pace I needed to go Sub-3 and to beep when my heart rate touched the PR deflection line.

I tried it out in London 2004 or 2005 and there was a small catch to this logic. Sooner or later your heart rate hits the deflection line, and you slow down to bring it back under, but then you aren't running fast enough to go Sub-3 so the too slow beeper starts. You will need to speed up again but then the heart rate monitor starts beeping, and before you know it you are trapped between the beeps. Sooner or later it's either death by pulse rate or death by road speed. Either way its death!

Maybe the simpler answer is to eat more carbs before the race. Three bowls of pasta instead of two. But not according to Page 16 "The most important source of energy for performing intensely in sports is carbohydrates. Carbohydrates can supply the most energy per time unit. Whenever the intensity of the exertion is lower the burning of fat begins to play an important role". So, more carbs then! "A 400-meter runner gets their energy supplied via the burning up of carbohydrates. For a cyclist or marathon runner in which endurance is most important the burning up of fat is used". So not three bowls of pasta then! "For well-trained persons the quantity of carbohydrates is about 700-800 gm. This quantity is sufficient to last for 60-90 minutes of intense exercise.

If carbohydrates are not replenished during this time.... this is the moment the athlete will suffer from getting the bonks". Aha, so eat as much pasta as you want but it will only fuel 60 minutes or so of intense exertion. Unless you are within an hour of the finish it's not a good idea to be going above the deflection line. The only way you are going to do this is to increase your base capacity to increase that deflection line to run faster without crossing it too early in the race.

If science is your thing then this is the book for you. I found a reader review, and this sums it up quite well.

"I've had this book many years ago and had to re buy to refresh my memory. Great book but you will get bogged down with graphs and techy information. The jist of the text is that if you train smart with your heart rate monitor you will give yourself optimum work outs. This is done by finding your lactate threshold. This is where you basically produce lactate acid at a given heartbeat say 150 bpm. This number will and can be raised over time by running at that pace when your body becomes lactate tolerant. In other words, your leg muscles that get sore and fatigued when you go for a run will disappear over time."

8.   Trailwalker 2004 - Mystic Chris

Within the new spirit of 'forget marathons and try something else' came the chance to walk or run an event called Trailwalker. Billed as the course that the Gurkhas' use to keep fit this was a 100k cross country event starting at The Queens Country Park near Petersfield and ending at Brighton Racecourse via The South Downs. My colleague Chris had introduced me to the event, and I thought why not.

The challenge was simple, walk, jog, or run with a team of four in under thirty hours with a support crew who would be parked up here and there along the way with a car full of food and drink. Life was now more about Ironman and extreme distance races vs a Sub-3 marathon challenge which seemed beyond me anyway having tried for fourteen years or more to do it. We weren't planning to run it all the way, but we weren't walking it all the way either and maybe we could finish within a decent time.

This was a team event so the individual selfishness of a marathon could take a back seat here and maybe the objective was to get us all through it. Chris, his brother, another friend, and me set off and his partner and other partners acted as support crew. It turned out to be a great day in great conditions, with great company and we all crossed the line together in 14:55 which, coincidentally, is the amount of time it can take to do an Ironman. Perfect base training.

Chris had run his first marathon in 2001, the year I had returned from working in the USA, and we spent the next ten years or so as work colleagues at the same firm. We weren't running buddies, but we sometimes ran the same race, and kept tabs on each other's stories, compared notes and kept up with each other's progress.

Whereas I was, or had been, on a quest for Sub-3, Chris was pursuing Sub-4 in the hope that he would move to chasing Sub-3. He asked me one day if I could help him with Sub-3. I told him to come back when he had figured out how to go Sub-3:30. That may sound arrogant, but I figured I would get a similar response if I asked someone how to go Sub-2:30.

Chris deserves a special place in this book, and I contacted him recently to clarify all of the things he used to do to get entries to races and to make himself faster. You might find some of his techniques useful, and somewhat eccentric at times, but above all you will find some of them funny and bizarre.

Like me, Chris used to find it hard to get an entry to the London Marathon. Whereas I would simply go and run it anyway and get taken off the course by the finish bouncers, Chris would create multiple pseudonyms and variations of his name and submit multiple entries. Not so long ago, the marathon organisers had a condition of guaranteeing a place following three, or five years, or so of rejections and Chris managed to get ballot places based on that condition.

Chris figured with multiple entries he would stand a better chance over time. He was a salesman and saw this as building an 'entry pipeline'. Some years he ended up getting more than one acceptance and had to get a deferral for the following year. It seemed over-complicated to me, but it worked for him. I had applied for the ballot one way or another for twenty years in a row, or more, and every year was the same. Thanks, but no thanks, and here's a new training jacket to let everyone know you didn't get in. We now both agree there is more to a fulfilling running life than the London Marathon.

Chris is not Mystic Chris for his race entry system. He is Mystic Chris for all of the strange things he used to come up with to run faster. His initial idea was Creatine Supplement and for his first race he mixed a big bag and ran with it on his back. The bag broke due to the constant pounding and he was left running with a deep red sticky fluid running down his legs. He moved on to energy gels and would be carrying a tool-belt full of them. He would mix the gels with pro-plus tablets and Nurofen in the hope that a combination of energy and pain suppression might somehow do the trick.

One year I bumped into him at the London Marathon registration Expo, and he was wearing magnets he had just bought from one of the stands. He had a necklace and two bracelets on, and other gadgets stuck to his legs. I was becoming concerned about his state of mind. They were called Phiten!

'Phiten necklaces contain the unique Aquatitan relaxation technology. Simply by wearing these products, your body can feel relaxed and refreshed. Phiten-Health-Necklaces are an indispensable item to support relief of stress, tension, and fatigue in our modern lives'.

I will leave you to decide how effective these might be to get you Sub-3. He tried Compression Shorts and "Running Orthotics" which are high-end in-soles for shoes costing £300 a pair which he managed to get on the company's health plan. None of these things were getting him to Sub-4 let alone Sub-3. He tried various forms of foot massage treatment days before a race, along with aromatherapy treatment again covered under the company's health plan. He paid £500 to learn how to use gravity to help him run faster! He explained how this was supposed to work.

"The technique was to lean forward like you were falling and harness the power of gravity like you were falling downhill! This led me to running around a 400M track with others, where at some point, one or more of us would fall over like toddlers onto the track! Apparently if you get it right, it is effortless, but I felt like I was David Carradine in the 1970s Kung Fu TV series, trying to learn to walk on rice paper. It was all very Karate Kid a sort of wash-on-wash-off kind of training. I left somewhat puzzled and with less money!"

He tried a more progressive form of gym training. "I paid £800 to go to a gym in Chiswick where they put you on a huge treadmill, twice the height of a normal one, and increase the incline and speed until you could take no more! The safety part was a chap with his hand at your back, which was like my grandad putting his arm out when braking heavily in the early 1970s. I watched one chap run so hard he was sick, and then I realised it was a regular thing. They also put me on an arm machine to cycle my arms, the theory being to drive the arms to drive the legs. The downside of that is that I got in my company car and pulled out onto the A4, indicating as I went. I lost all control of my arms and pulled the indicator stalk off like a second-rate David Banner turning into the Hulk (I was green from all the running to exhaustion and being sick). I had to explain to HR how and why I had broken the car."

Chris even tried sleep hypnosis where positive messages are subliminally pumped into you during sleep in the hope you will wake up as Steve Cram rather than Mystic Chris.

Eventually, Chris worked out that weight was the key factor. At 5' 7" weighing 75kg he realised he was on the high end of the weight spectrum and needed to be lighter to go faster.

I was sitting in my office soon after Chris had returned from a sales trip to the USA. He came in with a pensive look on his face and a cunning plan, cautiously looking around the rest of the office to make sure no-one was watching.

He closed the door and announced something he had found to help running performance. I was expecting a bag of syringes and weird looking liquids or something. He pulled a clear plastic bag from his pocket with a dozen bright blue pills in it and offered them over.

Now I don't do pills for leisure or sport and back then not for other purposes either, so this had to be good, or I might need to call the authorities. It turned out Chris had managed to source some fast diet pills whilst over in the USA. According to Chris, they were not available in the UK. He had ordered them over the phone from his hotel room and had explained he was shorter and heavier than he actually was so they would agree to sell to him and deliver to his hotel.

This is why he is Mystic Chris!

I don't know how many he had bought, but he was offering me a dozen of them at no charge. He had done the research. The secret of rapid weight loss is these tablets. He went through the rationale that they dissolve fat immediately and your body is only left with the good stuff and not the bad stuff. I put the bag in my desk drawer where I would re-find it ten years later when I left the company. I did try one the day he gave them to me. I felt a bit dizzy throughout the day in the office, so I passed on taking anymore.

Having re-connected with Chris recently, I brought the pill-popping era up, and asked whether he had persevered with it, given he had bought quite a large quantity of them. Yes, he said, and that he had shared them with friends and family who were interested in losing weight the "easy way", but there was a difficult side effect.

The main problem with them, he said, was the rapid conversion of fat to "cooking oil". It was best not to eat anything fatty as the tablets would convert it to a dark black oily liquid that was beyond difficult to retain, and harder still to remove as a stain.

One of his friends ruined a set of garden furniture and Chris still owns a sofa with cushions that can only be used one side up. Chris was kind enough to offer details of the tablets for anyone who wants to adopt this go faster tactic.

"Orlistat, sold under the brand name Xenical among others, is a medication used to treat obesity. Its primary function is preventing the absorption of fats from the human diet by acting as a lipase inhibitor, thereby reducing caloric intake."

Chris did own up to another tactic so far not shared with anyone, and he had to go into another room to confess his sins over the phone.

Our company annual sales conferences were always held in the first two weeks of April on a Thursday after year-end and typically days before the London Marathon. Chris took the opportunity to book a combined flotation and colonic irrigation treatment on the Friday afternoon while travelling home from the conference.

One treatment was for relaxation, the other to drop a few pounds, literally. He turned up at the start line a few pounds lighter and more relaxed than normal but Sub-4 was still not to be.

Chris eventually moved on to a more conventional from of weight loss and got his weight down from 73kg to 62kg which is the rock bottom low-end for someone 5' 7". He finally broke his Sub-4 target at this weight and achieved his marathon PB of 3:47:52.

Maybe the secret to all of this is weight. My PB was in 2008 when my weight was at its lowest, due to the amount of training for Ironman. Modest Martin (see Chapter 27) also cited weight as a significant key to his PB.

Chris is one of the most eccentric people I know and has tried dozens of different tactics to run faster over time. He has completed over seventy-five marathons and not come close to a Sub-3 but had he sussed earlier that weight is the key to speed then he could have done it. It sounds simple and maybe it is as simple as that.

9.   London Marathon 2005

Run less run faster

By London 2005, Ironman had fully taken over from marathon running in terms of interest and priority. Over the previous two years since Ironman Switzerland, I had completed three or four Ironman's and as many 'half irons' (aka 70.3) and was sharing training time between swim, bike and run. I was probably running less than at any time in the past fourteen or fifteen years but feeling stronger and fitter. I was keeping a daily record of swim, bike, and run activity, and averaging around three hours a week running and six hours a week cycling through long cycle trips at weekends.

My London Marathon time (2004) was a PB at 3:15:50. I think this qualified me for a Good for Age place in 2005. This was the year after Rhino Guy had attempted a Sub-4 'Rhino Marathon' and narrowly missed it at 4:20. He had spent the winter training in Hyde Park in a Rhino costume from the Circle of Life show. Trust me, those Rhino suits are as heavy as armour. It was also the year that Paula Radcliffe would run a 2:17. So could this be it? Had the switch to triathlon improved my chances of a Sub-3 or would this be another failed attempt, like every other time since 1990.

The night before the race was Rhino Guy's 40th birthday party. The challenge to stay out late despite the race the following day was thrown down and duly accepted, as was the constant delivery of drinks and shots by Rhino Guy throughout the night. As usual a forfeit and bet were required and a spread bet was created whereby, I would owe him £10 for every minute over three hours, and he would owe me £5 for every minute under three. Clearly no risk for me because, as always, there could be no chance I will run slower than three hours. For Rhino Guy this was important too. He had Sub-3'd two years earlier and had held overall marathon bragging rights with that time ever since. My Sub-3 was not something he was hoping for so was keeping me out late, and with as many shots as possible to dampen my chances, literally.

I was getting faster despite running less. Two years ago, I ran the normal 3:32, so no change there. A year ago, and this was cut down by fifteen minutes to finish in 3:15. Now with three Ironman finishes under my belt confidence was running high, despite a late night out and half a dozen tequila shots.

The first 10K of the race was looking good at 40:22 with a smattering of club runners around me, so I was still in fast company. The clock at halfway was showing 1:27:07 and I had never been this far below 1:30 at the half before and, more importantly, I was still feeling strong. Surely this is on.

Some people say the race doesn't really start until you get into the teen miles and for those who know the London course, will also know that at halfway you are turning away from London and out towards Canary Wharf. There is a four, or five, mile stretch where you need to dig in hard before you turn for home and head back towards the city with about eight or nine miles to hang on in there.

London has a two-mile stretch going out to Canary Wharf between mile-13 and mile-15 and coming back from Canary Wharf between mile-20 and mile-22 where you are running opposite runners going in the other direction. On the way out you might see the elite men and women coming the other way which is both inspiring to see them so far ahead and demoralising because you are miles away from that point in the race. On the way back, however, you have the main field still running out to Canary Wharf and you know they are looking at you wishing they were where you are.

From here, there are still four or five miles to go, and it starts to become clear you are slowing down as other runners are starting to pass you. This is one of the dark places you will have to go to if you are going to do this. You have come this far, you are 'on-track' but the demons of doubt are beginning to circle around you.

Soon it's Blackfriars and the run down to the tunnel at the start of the Embankment, and a nasty little, short hill which brings you to the 24-mile mark. Two to go. Sixteen, seventeen minutes inside Sub-3. That's eight-and-a-half-minute mile pace plus the extra bit at the end (the 0.2 of the 26.2 added to the marathon distance by Queen Alexandra at the 1908 Olympics by moving the start to the lawn at Windsor Castle so that the young royals could watch it from their nursery. Thank you, Queen Alexandra!).

Surely, we (or I) are holding this pace. This must be in the bag. Another mile marker in sight but no, it's the 40K marker and just nine, or is it ten, minutes to spare. Two five-minute pace kilometres. This is it, come on! Every runner around you is nervously looking at their watch. They all know this is touch and go. They all have the same thing in mind. The turn at Big Ben, the marshals in long lines sending runners to the left of the road, then the right to filter you apart for the run to the finish. For some reason a '600 meters to go' sign shows up as you near the right turn to Buckingham Palace.

A lap and a half of a running track, that's all there is. You try and sprint, but you can't. You think you are sprinting, but you are merely maintaining deterioration. Running zombies are all around you, all faced with the same reality and hoping maybe their chip time is behind the clock time, but for those who started on-the-line this is only worth seconds not minutes.

Rhino Guy and a team from The Serpentine Club were waiting at the top of the small hill towards Buckingham Palace, looking straight down towards the last but one turn just a few hundred metres from the finish.

Rumour has it that Rhino Guy had said "if he doesn't come round that corner in the next 10 seconds its over". Ten seconds came and went. Fifteen, Twenty. Rhino Guy is counting his winnings and thinking his Sub-3 bragging rights are still intact when, one of the other Serpentines said, "There he is!"

This is going to be close. Very close. I can now hear the race commentator on the loudspeaker system as I pass by Buckingham Palace and turn onto The Mall. The finish is agonisingly further than I thought but I can see the clock and the grandstand full of people cheering and the clock still says "2" and for a split second it looks like it's on.

The minutes on the finish clock are showing 58 then 59 and the final seconds are evaporating before me. I tried one last time to sprint. I can see the athletes crossing the line ahead of me, arms aloft to celebrate their Sub-3. The race commentator starts counting down the clock to get the crowd cheering and I realise I am about to become the first of the losers as the "3" clicks ahead of me and I cross the line in 3.00.33.

Like coming 4th in a Championship race, you just missed out. "Nice try", "great time", PB, "can't believe you ran that fast", "you must be pleased", but no, you are not a Sub-3 runner. You can't excuse away thirty-three seconds. Maybe the clock was wrong? I may as well as have finished 3:20+ like all the other times. If it were 1990 I would still be required to wear that dress. I walked to the kit lorries passing other athletes all congratulating themselves and swopping Sub-3 stories no doubt.

I boarded the tube, people were saying well done, but it was time to forget and move on. Just another attempt. I'm not getting any younger. Maybe next year.

Rhino Guy was elated at my failed attempt as his bragging rights were still intact. I asked how he knew I couldn't have sprinted that last bit but he knows, like I know, you simply can't. There is no sprint finish, there's nothing left. It was as good as a miss three miles back.

So, 2005, and fifteen years of trying was another year that was not to be.

Or was it? London is not the be all and end all of marathons. With thirty-three seconds to find surely now was the time to find it. After a few hours sulking over what could and should have been in London 2005 I opened the laptop and started searching for another race somewhere in the UK that wouldn't clash with Ironman races. Nottingham? Dublin?

10.   Dublin Marathon 2005
Maybe this time!

Here we go again. I remembered a footballer friend of mine had recently run Dublin in a time of 3:22 having set out for a Sub-3. Familiar story. He said it was a good course and felt he could have done better. As Dublin is in October this might be the perfect timing, having completed two Ironman's since the London Marathon in April, as well as the Nottingham marathon a month earlier as a warm-up.

The race wasn't full and getting an entry was straight forward. Dublin was familiar territory having been to several rugby internationals in the 90's. I checked in to Buswells Hotel in the city centre just a 20-minute walk to the start at Fitzwilliam Square. The race is on the last Sunday of October, so it works to arrive on Saturday, run on Sunday and stay for the Monday Bank Holiday.

October meant perfect weather conditions for me, three or four degrees lower than perfect running conditions for everyone else. There was a breeze and a light drizzle before the start, so a possibility of cramp but better than the prospect of any sunshine.

The start area wasn't packed so getting a place close to the front runners was easy, even though I knew a lot of them would pass me early on. On paper the course is 'mostly flat' which is shorthand for a few hills here and there. A course review guide reads:

"Elevation: The course is mostly flat with a few hills throughout. However, there is one long drag between miles 21-22 that can break your heart. It's not that it's very steep, it's just very long and gradual and occurs at a point in the race where you might be hanging on for dear life!"

I never spend time memorising a particular course or driving round it on a reconnaissance mission as the only thing that matters on race day is how nervous you are feeling, how hot it is and whether you can get some breakfast down before the race. The rest is in the hands of the gods.

The plan, as always, was to make halfway with time on the clock (Sub 1:30) and hope to be feeling as strong as when you started. From there it's just hold pace and hope. I noted the hill at mile 21-22 and that it looked downhill and flat from there, so I aimed to be at the top of that hill by 2:30 for there to be any chance of a Sub-3.

The first two miles are pretty much downhill, building a false sense of security before the entry to Phoenix Park and a gradual climb of about 200 meters to mile-7 which took its toll on my pace, but I was still feeling good and the reward of a three mile downhill to mile-10 and out the other side of the park re-established a sense of belief that this was on.

A nasty steep little climb to mile-11 took the smile of my face and put me back into the red zone. Then a two-mile flat section, empty of spectators, took us to the all-important halfway mark and a check on progress. The clock showed 1:28, and some, and the sudden reality of another failed attempt stated to run through my mind.

London just six months earlier had been a minute, or two, faster than this at halfway and that had ended in tears at 3:00:33 so this was not looking good with the hill at mile 21-22 still to come. Panic was starting to set in, but any runner will tell you there's not much you can do about this. Slow down, and it's over, speed up and risk bonking later, it's still over, holding pace, seems a good idea but you start getting slower without realising.

Tragically, the road started to rise slightly from mile-13 which should have been curtains but it was short lived, and the road flattened out again just after mile-14. I was able to settle down for the next three or four miles and maybe, just maybe, I was still on schedule. A blessing came at mile-17 as the road gradually declined through and past mile-20 so surely I had gained some time, or at least held pace.

Everything now was about running to the pace of your body, not your watch, which can't help you. Switch off the crowd, forget the course clocks (as its too difficult to work out past half-way anyway) and tune into the Sub-3 soundtrack and find something, anything, to hold pace.

Stay with runners next to you for as long as you can. Hold on to their feet. Another two songs and another mile. A quick drink at an aid station but not too much. Just hang on in there. And then the hill. As advertised, it's not very steep but it is long. How bloody long? Initially it's steeper than expected but it doesn't look long and then it suddenly turns right ahead of you. Then back round to the left and you can see the top of it into the distance.

Remember, it's all downhill from the top? Well downhill and then flat. I don't know precisely where the top is from memory, either the start or end of Foster's Avenue but I think the 22-mile marker was the point of hope. I glanced at my watch which was showing 2:28 or 2:29, or whatever, but with four miles still to go and just over 7-minute mile pace to hold to do it. Surely this wasn't going to be another thirty second miss like London. The games' not over don't throw the towel in now.

I remember the left turn at the top of the hill onto the big dual carriageway that had been cordoned off for the race that went on for half a mile or so before the right tun past a golf course and left onto Merrion Road. The run through Ballsbridge and past the Registration Centre where I had thought to myself the day before "this time and place tomorrow will be judgement day".

At mile-24 I glanced at my watch one last time. I had seventeen or eighteen minutes still in the bank which felt like a decent cushion, but I was flagging fast with 2.2 miles to go and that last 0.2 miles could make the difference again.

I found myself running beside a woman who had crept up from behind me. She was clearly struggling like me, but she was holding pace, and I was slipping. She had a club running shirt on, so I clung to her praying for that finish line. There are more corners and turns and is this ever going to end? The crowds were getting deeper and louder as I came up Northumberland Street and into Mount Street but still the finish line is "just around the corner" like the corner before that and the corner before that.

I managed to find some last-minute energy and pulled ahead of the woman having said to her "hold in there, you're nearly there". Empty words of course if that bloody clock clicks three. Then it was in sight. The finish gantry about 200 yards ahead but I couldn't see the clock so sod the watch just hang on, hold on, stumble on, and get over that line wherever it was.

The clock said "2" something I was certain of it, and I checked back as I crossed the line to see it had just gone 2:59. I started welling up, as I am a sentimental old sod, and the enormity of it what had just happened was beginning to dawn on me.

I looked back again, and I could see the woman I had shared those last few miles with coming towards the finish. I shouted and shouted at her to go for it, and she crossed in 2:59:30 or something similar and I gave her a big tearful hug. We had both just done something I, at least, had dreamt of doing since those silly bet days of 1990.

Fifteen years and some later, the Sub-3 curse had finally been broken. I didn't really care what the minutes and seconds were I just wanted that "2" and something title. My finish time was in fact 2:58:48 and I can't tell you what a feeling that was. Collecting your medal, your goody bag, walking back to the hotel, through the spectators, knowing you are a Sub-3 marathon runner.

An after-race Guinness would never taste as good as it would now.

When you finish an Ironman, they announce everyone as they cross the line "John Smith, you are an Ironman". I wanted someone to announce, "Andy Bass, you are a Sub-3 man".

I knew how those who were finishing just behind us were feeling right now. I watched a handful of them crossing the line in 3:00:10, 3:00:20 and so-on while I was gathering my breath.

There's nothing worse than a near miss, surely there was something you could have done to find that 10 seconds, that 20 seconds, even that minute but you can't.

So, Dublin 2005 was that special day for me, and it will always hold pride of place in my heart. I returned four more times in 2009-12 to run the Dublin marathon and made it a perfect five with a Sub-3 every time. Every year we stayed at Buswells Hotel and every year we got laced up on Guinness and a banquet to celebrate.

Sadly, a work colleague from Dublin had passed away with cancer at a very young age and for a few years a crew of us from the company ran for her charity and in her memory. The company generously doubled whatever amount we had raised.

She had vowed to beat cancer and watch us run but sadly she didn't make it, so we made Dublin a "Run-4-Janice" event for two or three years in a row. Her family and friends would come and join us in Buswells after the race.

RIP Janice, God bless and a special shout out to Tom, Ollie and Owen, the Run-4-Janice Team. Tom was a hard-core rower, so he was used to explosive and endurance racing.

For Ollie and Owen who were Ireland based this would be their first ever marathon and it would be a special time for them to get over the finish line. Between us we raised over £30,000 for a charity close to her heart.

On a side note, the 1:28 half split in 2005 was the slowest half of all my Sub-3 finishes and I am not someone who can handle neutral or negative splits. Others can, but this is a key part of the race tactic that you need to understand (See Chapter 28).

11. Great Wall Marathon 2006
Sub-4 is Sub-3

The Great Wall of China Marathon is on every marathon runner's bucket list. It's not easy to enter and harder to run. There are 5,164 steps to climb up to, across, and down off the wall over the course of the race. These are not diddy step size they are steep and high and the final climb onto the wall leaves you literally crawling.

Part of the run is through dusty villages on hilly terrain, and a couple of falls at speed are par for the course when the rocks catch your feet and take you down hard.

The race guide for The Great Wall of China Marathon tells you to add 40% to your normal marathon time when setting a target. So, assuming a 'new' normal time of 2:50 plus 40% would mean a target time of 3.58 so Sub-4 on The Great Wall is equivalent to a Sub-3 elsewhere.

I researched the results history of the race over a twenty-year period from 1999 to 2019. Of the 5,000 or so people that have run it in those years, less than eighty have completed the course in under four hours.

Having organised a business trip to China to take twenty leading state school UK heads to create twinned partnerships with schools in Beijing, I managed to bunk off on the Friday night and be driven down to the wall for the start of the race the next day.

This is not the tourist part of the wall, and it is a few hours' drive out of Beijing. Getting the right papers and entrance to the race was all done via an agency, who were managing the school trip on the company's behalf, so it was an absolute bonus to get to do this.

The Huang Ya hotel by the race start was sparse to say the least, not much better than a cell in Alcatraz. It had about a dozen rooms, no locks on the doors, curtains hanging off the rails and a combined walk-in shower/toilet. Well, this is a poorer part of China, and it was better to stay over than being bused down from Beijing at the crack of dawn.

The pre-race set up was bizarre. A few hundred runners milling around inside The Great Wall Fort in Yin Yang Square at the foot of Huang YaGuan entrance to the Great Wall. There was a fortress garden where the race would start.

Musicians in a truck straight out of the film The Grapes of Wrath turned up and proceeded to play a variety of tunes with a Michael Jackson look-a-like wandering around with a cane. He didn't seem to be doing any singing and he was flanked by a couple of other people dressed in odd costumes.

The band played several vaguely familiar pop songs as the runners arrived on coaches that had presumably made the three-hour trip from Beijing, and we proceeded to the start area and began to warm up.

The marathon start was two waves of a hundred or so runners starting five minutes apart. The first five kilometres were on a winding road leading up to the base of The Great Wall and where we would be climbing steps for the first time onto the top of it.

I set off with the leaders of Wave 2 and we soon began eating our way through the tail end of the Wave 1 runners. The first section of the wall wasn't overly horrendous, just a few hundred steps up to get onto it then a series of lower steps running across the wall.

The feeling of running somewhere completely unique was awesome and the views were spectacular. I had a throw away camera and took snaps as we ran. The first section of the wall takes you through several towers with names like The Widows Tower and The Blind Tower and I expected David Carradine to turn up any minute with a red-hot urn from a Shaolin temple.

There are fifteen towers on the first stretch of the wall and by half-way through the first section it felt as though we had caught most of Wave 1, except for any of the faster ones who were out of sight but had a 5-minute gap to maintain.

You run 5k or so along the wall before doing a lap of Yin Yang square, still on top of it, and then you drop back down via a few hundred steps before the course takes you off on the main village roads, across a rickety bridge or two into Duanzuang village, through Chedaoyu village and Qingshaning village before you head back on the return road, loop across another rickety bridge and start the run back to Yin Yang Square.

The villages were sparse with locals and livestock both wondering who and why people were running through their towns and villages. There were some very steep dusty and rocky road downhill sections where I came down hard as I was running too fast, and my head couldn't keep up with my feet. I lost my camera, my drinks bottle, and a bit of skin on my hands and knees but was feeling quite strong.

The route headed back to the Fort and at around twenty miles I passed one of the Wave 1 front runners who had dropped back. I asked him how many ahead and he said three, so a podium finish was now on the cards, and I pressed on.

Running into the fort I caught up with another Wave 1 runner and given, the 5-minute start gap, I am now firmly in 3rd place. I heard the commentator say here comes 3rd and 4th so that seemed to confirm my thinking. From the Fort you run the first section of the wall again, but the other way round and the climb up is hell on earth.

Over a thousand steps all at different heights which left me literally crawling up the final hundred steps or so. The 4th placed guy dropped well behind me so all to do now was a flat run across the wall, through a few turrets and towers, and up and down a few hundred lower height steps.

As I emerged from the final tower, I saw a race photographer in front of me and I still have the picture of me holding up three fingers as I ran past him, not knowing how far ahead the other two were.

My excitement was short lived. As I turned to go back down the steps to the final 5k back to the finish, a guy from the Wave 2 start appeared from nowhere and went past me at pace. I dug in to hold on, but he had the measure of me, and I finished a hundred meters behind him to discover I had come 4th. A consolation time of 03:57:24, with just four of us going Sub-4 that year.

Back at the Fort and Yin Yang square there was an hour or two to soak in the enormity of, and privilege of, having the opportunity to run this race. I bought a couple of T-Shirts, took some photos of the runners still yomping their way up to the final section of the wall, said thank you to Michael Jackson and the band that was still playing and got a car back to Beijing for tea, medals and a few well-earned beers.

The Great Wall Marathon was duly ticked off the marathon bucket list with an 'honorary' Sub-3.

12. August 2006 A Norseman Black and Zombie Hill

Just as The Great Wall Marathon is on every runner's bucket list, so the Norseman is on every Ironman bucket list. The Norseman is not a branded Ironman but is Ironman distance with a twist. As you might expect it is in Norway. Back in the early days, an Ironman was a mass start mad dash into the sea or a lake, and you were in a human washing machine for as long as it took for the race to spread out. Modern day Ironman has a rolling start so they can reduce the risk of drowning and accommodate more entrants.

The Norseman starts before dawn with a car ferry trip two miles out in a Norwegian fjord, and a jump from the back of the ferry into the cold dark waters below. The race is limited to a few hundred athletes and their supporters and after the athletes have been 'dropped off' (literally) the ferry returns to shore taking the support crews back with it to prepare for the bike transition as the athletes start to emerge from the water.

In 2006 I entered relatively late and there were still plenty of slots available. Today, like the London Marathon, race entry is down to a ballot and getting a place is unlikely. In 2022, there were over 4,500 entries for just two hundred places. Three months earlier I had committed the ultimate sin of a DNF at Ironman France in Nice. The Norseman was a chance for redemption.

Why are we digressing into Ironman stories when this book is about going Sub-3 in a marathon? Well going Sub-3 in a marathon delivers legendary status so imagine what status a Sub-3 marathon within an Ironman delivers. Although, having never Sub-3'd an Ironman marathon, nor come remotely close, there is another reason to include this race, Zombie Hill, and a Norseman Black.

There is no feed station support throughout the entire Norseman race except for a table of drinks at the foot of Zombie Hill, which is 25k into the marathon, and a water barrel at about 30k, halfway up Zombie Hill. You must bring your own support person or crew to a Norseman, who can follow you in a car throughout the race to stop at pre-determined points to take on drinks or food.

My seventy-year-old father had agreed to be my support. Having landed in Oslo, we drove for three hours to the run finish to check out the course, and to leave the bike box at the hotel where we would be staying the following evening, should we both make it to the finish. From there we drove the reverse run and bike course through 140 miles of the Hardinger valley to the start of the race at a large fjord in Eidford.

The enormity of the bike course climbs, with over 5,000 meters of climbing started to set in as we drove. The huge expectation and responsibility I had put on my father to record and remember suitable stop points along the way, also set in.

We aimed for a handful of places where there were small grocery stores that had ice. My father's main instructions were to get ice wherever he could, as warm drinks for me are, a complete no-no. After the 2.4-mile swim (1:18 time), a quick change from wetsuit into cycling gear and onto the 112-mile hilly bike course for almost eight hours of cycling. From there, another change to running gear and the start of the marathon, after almost nine-and-half hours on the go.

Although the marathon should be my strong point it is typically anything but, as I am normally so wasted by the time I get to it, that its touch and go as to whether I will even finish.

There are no finisher medals for the Norseman. There are three T-shirt options, one is no T-shirt at all, if you don't finish. The second is a white finisher T-shirt if you don't make the 33k run mile mark within the cut-off time of 13:15 (you are then required to run the final 10K back to the finish hotel along a flat road). The third is the coveted Norseman Black T-Shirt, where you make the 33k cut-off within the time, and are certified fit and healthy enough to attempt the 10k ultra-steep climb to the top of Gaustatoppen, 1,900 meters above sea level.

So, the marathon is 25k flat at sea level, then an 8k steep climb to the 33k mark at about 1,500 meters, known as "Zombie Hill", then a further 2k flat, then a 7k climb up a very rocky steep cliff to the finish.

You are required to have the support crew member go with you on the final ascent, but it was too big of a risk for my elderly father, so I tagged on to another runner and his crew. I surprisingly flew the first 25k of the run. Everything felt great and it was probably my best Ironman marathon ever for that first 25k.

My father was great, he kept the car stocked up with lots of different drinks and ice and I managed to fuel up four or five times during the first part of the run.

You can see Gaustatoppen mountain rising high into the distance from the start of the run and at 25k you make a left turn for the climb to the 33k marker. At the start of the climb someone has chalked on the road in massive letters "Welcome to Zombie Hill".

By the time you make it to the 33k marker you are walking like a Zombie trying to make sure the marshals won't rule you unfit to press on for a Black T-Shirt finish. The road up to the 33k marker is narrow, windy, and steep and there is nowhere for support cars to stop so you are on your own.

There are no aid stations except for one large water barrel halfway up with WATER written on it. My father was proudly at the 33k marker and was as elated as I was when they passed me as fit and OK to go on. He drove the next two or three kilometres to the start of the steep rocky climb. We parted company and he went back to the hotel for a well-earned sleep.

When you reach the top, there are no cheering crowds just a guy with a clip board who ticks your name off and you can get a beer or some soup or both. It is a No.1

Ironman bucket list to finish and, whereas there are probably now hundreds of thousands of people who have completed an Ironman worldwide, there are probably only a few thousand that own a Norseman Black.

At the top of the mountain, I phoned Rhino Guy and gave him ten guesses where I was sitting right now. He struggled for a while until I told him I was wearing a black T-shirt and then it clicked.

He has since got his own, and his wife has too, having won the race a few years later. The T-shirts are awarded the following day back down at the finish hotel. Every finisher is called out one by one and the shirt is awarded to them individually just like getting a rugby Lion's Jersey for the first test.

It is a special race and a special marathon. Despite a fast first 25k of the run at Sub 3:30 pace my final run time was 5:17:47, Zombie Hill and the final climb must have taken me over three hours.

13. San Francisco Marathon 2007

Son of San

A company I used to work for provided an Executive Training budget and within reason I could chose my own course at any University anywhere worldwide. After a reasonably extensive search I settled on a week-long Strategy and Leadership course at Stanford University.

As we had previously lived in California it made sense for my family to fly out with me and spend a week in Southern California with friends and then fly up to San Francisco at the end of the week to meet me. Perfect.

By complete and utter chance, the timing of the course coincided with the San Francisco Marathon. As coincidental as the trip to China coinciding with The Great Wall Marathon and future business trips to Tokyo coinciding with the Tokyo Marathon.

My eldest son had recently turned twelve and there was a half marathon happening at the same time as the full marathon. The flexible organisers were happy for me and my son to start in the same wave together.

The plan was for my wife and my youngest son to cheer us on through the start and 'past Pier 39' (see Stereophonics on Sub-3 soundtrack) and to get to the end of the half marathon where they would somehow find him finishing in amongst the tens of thousands of other runners doing the half. I would carry on and finish the full and meet them back at Pier 39 near the finish.

Simple, what could go wrong! Well other than worrying halfway through the race whether he would get lost at the finish and be picked up by a trafficking gang never to be seen again, it seemed like a good idea and a massive father-son bonding moment.

The start time was ridiculously early as they were closing the Golden Gate bridge for us to run across. Imagine that, running the San Francisco Marathon right behind your son and crossing the Golden Gate Bridge over and back. Despite there being little chance of a Sub-3, this was a special moment in my sporting journey.

My son was a little eager and when the hooter went off for the start of our wave, he shot off at such a pace he led the entire wave down the San Fran Pier 39-37 sea front, and I couldn't keep up with him.

Eventually I got to him and made him slow down and he held out for at least nine or ten miles before he started flagging a bit, but it was a memory for life as he turned left to the half marathon finish, and I turned right for the second half of the full.

Yes, my wife was there somewhere and found him – he finished in 2:04 and won his age group though there were only four runners in the race aged twelve!

My son is now in his twenties and has run a few marathons and completed a few Ironman races and has a Sub-3 in his sights. Having run the London Vitality half a few years ago in 1:35, completely exhausted he realised why the Sub-3 challenge is the holy grail for amateur runners.

He has since, and so far, ran a 3:15, but like his old man this is a background hobby for him, not something worth giving up drink and life for.

Much of my time now is spent organising and supporting him at various events, driving him to start lines, picking him up at finish lines and spending hours in cars, café's, and hotel rooms as main support crew. It seems like an individual sport, but for most of us it's a team event.

14. London Marathon 2008
Going Elite

This book is all about becoming a legend and going Sub-3. But what is beyond that? Well clearly unless you are Kipchogi or another professional athlete where it's all about podium finishes, world and national records, and Olympic qualification, then the next logical step for us amateurs is to make Elite status by going Sub-2.45.

This is a different ball game altogether. This is the point at which you qualify for the Elite Men's start for the London Marathon. Go Sub-2:45 and you will be on the front of Blue Start with the world's greatest marathon runners. You will literally be lining up with the GOATs of marathon running.

Having cracked Sub-3 on several occasions, and with the benefits of Ironman training, I set my sights on Elite status.

The 2008 London Marathon was the last time Good for Age athletes started at the front of the Green Start. This may have been partly my fault after an altercation with the cast of EastEnders, other TV luvvies, and an Olympic champion here and there. This was to become my fastest ever marathon, and my most memorable one, all because of 'Elmbridge Guy'.

The Good for Age runners were gathered behind the second rope at the start line. I found myself standing in the front row of the race and going through my final preparations like peeing in a bottle, and over most of my hands, wearing a black bin liner to keep warm, usual cap, sunglasses, and making final adjustments to the MP3 player to make sure the headphones would stay in my ears and not keep falling out.

I asked the guy next to me "What time are you going for?" "2:45" he said "You?" "Uh yeah 2:45", I said having no plan to do that. A minute or two later I asked him "What mile pace are you aiming for, 5:50/6 minute or something?" I enquired. "God No" he said "6:10". He seemed robotically certain of this race pace number, and I realised I was next to a proper runner given he had an Elmbridge running club shirt on and had a real plan.

My plan was to go out fast and hang on for the last thirteen miles. He said you must be no later than 2:30 at Mile-24 to do it and so I asked him if he didn't mind pacing me or mind me running next to or near him. I wouldn't be able to hear anything he might say during the race given the music, but he seemed very sure of how to pace a Sub-2:45.

This was my first time on the Green Start which unbeknown to me happened to also be the celebrity start. I was suddenly aware of Gordon Ramsay and James Cracknell (before they were Sub-3 runners) hanging around in a cordoned off area ahead of us, with a very posh toilet block vs the bog-standard Portaloo's we had all been queuing up for.

To my surprise, and dismay, we weren't at the start rope after all. There was another start rope about ten yards ahead of us on the real start line and a variety of C and D list celebrities started to appear in front of us a few minutes before the start. Bizarrely a group of African tribesmen with full length shields, traditional dress and spears appeared on the right side and started jumping up and down in a war type dance ritual. I think they had numbers on so must be running the race. Then, what I assumed was the cast of some TV series like EastEnders gathered in front of us, all chatting away like they were off on a 5K park run.

By the time all these vaguely familiar people had gathered they must have been five or ten deep between us, the Sub-2:45 line, and the actual Start line. Elmbridge Guy had told me the Green Start would be through narrow streets with parked cars for the first half mile or so hence he was starting at the front, or what now appeared to be the second front.

With one minute to go they removed the rope separating us from the celebs, and my first instinct was to get past them, vs mowing them down in the first fifty yards or so of the race. To go Sub-3 means a clear start, not weaving through traffic furniture and slow runners. The first mile is crucial to be up to speed, on pace and settled down.

The cast of EastEnders, or whoever they were, were not impressed as me and my new pacemaker and most of the others behind us barged to the front. It all got a bit heated but hey, we are not here for a five-hour jog. If it had been Frank Bruno, then maybe 'after you Frank', but I couldn't see anyone who looked like a professional boxer, Cracknell can probably handle himself, so we gave him a bit more room.

Elmbridge Guy was right about the start. The road out to where all the runners from the Red, Blue and Green starts would eventually meet up and merge together was tight and congested with cars, people and road furniture, but we got away in the front dozen or so runners, and we were up to speed straight away, and I didn't look back to see how the cast of EastEnders were doing. I settled down right behind Elmbridge Guy and to my surprise, the pace felt slow, even in that first half-a-mile or so. Surely this is not Sub-2:45 pace, I would normally be going quicker than this.

As we approached the first mile marker it still felt slow. As we came level with it, I glanced down at my watch. It said 6:10 on the nose. Exactly what Elmbridge Guy had said, and he looked across at me saying something, but I couldn't hear above the music, so I just put my thumb up.

This still felt slow, but I felt good and if this is what Sub-2:45 feels like then so far so good. At the 2-Mile marker I glanced again at my watch, and it showed 12:20, to the second. At the 3-Mile marker 18:30, at four miles 24:40 and so on.

We were metronomically on a 6:10 pace and this was the only run in my life where I had done this. I wasn't planning to attempt a Sub-2:45, for me Sub-3 was good enough, and had I attempted it under my own pace making I would probably have gone out at 5:50 pace and died in a ditch around the 18-mile marker.

By the 8-Mile marker I was struggling to calculate 6:10 pace in my head but I was still running right behind Elmbridge Guy. I left the pace making up to him as he seemed to have it down to a fine art. I was still feeling good, no parrots on either shoulder talking doubt into my mind, the mental parrot was asleep as was the physical one, neither were beginning to complain about anything.

There was something different about the runners around us. Remember this is Sub-2:45 pace and I started to realise that most of the runners around us had blue numbers on their backs. These were elite start runners, and they get issued with a front and back number that is blue on a white background. If you have ever gone to watch the London Marathon then you will see these runners coming through soon after the pro-men and women.

I thought our Good for Age numbers were something special, but we are now truly in fast and long company. There were groups of three and four runners pacing together, often with the same running club vests on like "Harrogate Harriers" or "Wimbledon Millers", predominantly gaunt, spindly men, as any women at this pace are bordering on professional.

There are no official pacemakers with their big time-flags guiding you in to help you, I guess they assume you have that covered. It was also very un-congested and there was lots of space around us. This, and London

2009, would be the only time I would experience being here. I wondered what Sub-2:30 must be looking like further ahead.

As we approached the feed station at the 12-Mile marker just before the right turn onto Tower Bridge I was still right behind Elmbridge Guy, and I still felt strong. I had also been disciplined at taking a sip of water at every feed station where I would normally skip it.

I briefly got caught up between drinking and concentrating and Elbridge Guy was suddenly about five to ten yards ahead of me. I kept calm, stayed with the pace as we went up the small rise to the middle of Tower Bridge and down the other side towards halfway. I realised I wasn't making any ground on him though he was still in sight just ahead.

I crossed halfway in 1:21:06, a time anyone running a half marathon would probably kill for, and the fastest half I have ever run. Surely, the wheels will be coming off soon and the dream will be over. Now for the boring teen miles and out to Canary Wharf. Elmbridge Guy is beginning to disappear into the distance. I can still see him on longer straights, but I finally lose sight of him around fifteen or sixteen miles and I am now on my own.

There is a decision to be taken here and now. Do I push hard to catch up and risk it all or do I stay on current pace, albeit slowing, I'm still feeling good and starting to think about a PB. I stay with pace. Maybe if I still feel good at Mile-20 I will go after it.

By Mile-24 reality started to set in as I clocked 2:31 and I remembered Elmbridge Guy had said it needed to be Sub 2:30 here. With two miles to go this is a slam dunk Sub-3 and now just a question of a PB.

The run into the finish is still a very vivid memory. 'Run' by Snow Patrol randomly came on the Sub-3 soundtrack just past Big Ben. Perfect. I wasn't flagging and crawling along, I wasn't in a dark place, I was still running at a good pace, and I crossed the line feeling strong with a PB of 2:46:30.

I had a whole new respect for those going Sub-2:45 and more so those ahead going Sub-2:30. Those are truly crazy times and come with God-like status for anyone who can run them.

I wondered what had become of Elmbridge Guy. I checked my split times when I got home later that evening after a celebratory night out with a few glasses of wine. I don't know if it was him for sure but someone running for that Club finished the race in 2:45:00. It must have been him! I suspect he would have preferred a second off that time. Without him I would probably have finished at my normal erratic pace somewhere between 2:50 and 2:59.

If you are going to attempt something this fast then you will need an Elmbridge Guy pace discipline. If, like me, you are prone to running too fast at the start then a Sub-2.45 is probably beyond you. You need to find a pacemaker or get expert at it yourself.

In the runners' pack for the following year's marathon was a letter for Good for Age Runner qualifiers. It started something along the lines of "Due to an altercation at the Green Start last year we have now moved the Good for Age Runners to the front of the Red Start".

So, for everyone who has ever started as Good for Age on the Red start vs the Green start, then you have me and Elmbridge Guy to thank for that.

Trust me the Red Start is better than the Green and they merge you ahead of the fun runners. Sincere apologies to all TV drama runners, African tribesmen, Gordon, and James if you got caught up in a bit of shoving and pushing that year, but Sub-3 runners should be taking start priority.

As a footnote James Cracknell ran 2:59:11 that year (2008) and I believe that was the first time he joined the Sub-3 Club and with just forty-eight seconds to spare. I checked out the Runners World Website from 2004, four years earlier, when James stated he wanted to run a Sub-3 Marathon in London 2005 (so a Sub-3 straight off the bat).

Here is a discussion thread from that site about Cracknell's initial Sub-3 statement which gets a few seasoned runners a bit agitated and animated. A few other celebrities and sports people get caught up in the debate.

"Is it just me or does anybody else find this attitude slightly patronising? He seems to be assuming that just

because he's good at one sport he'll be able to do this. I might be wrong, but I fancy the odds are against him. I guess being a rower he'll be a fairly hefty bloke and dragging any weight round sub 3 is gonna be tough. Plus, most of the weight and conditioning is going to be upper body and that won't help. Who thinks he'll do it - I vote no!"

"Good on him for actually putting down a target time. I'd be surprised if he made it but good luck to him. By stating a target time like this he's making it clear that he's going to be taking it really seriously which might be difficult mentally when he finds himself struggling behind those people who habitually run sub-3 but who still look the most unathletic of people."

"He'll know how Steve Redgrave got on in London (5hrs something?) and he's not stupid enough to assume it'll be easy."

"OK OK sorry! I wasn't really trying to diss him I just think a 3hr marathon is incredibly tough even for somebody with the right build. There are plenty of very good and experienced runners who would kill for a sub 3hr marathon."

"Approximate times (from memory) for sports people running marathons. Steven Redgrave - 5hrs something, Richard Dunwoody - 3hr 10, Seb Coe - 2:58, Steve Cram - 2:30, Some top swimming chap whose name escapes me (Adrian Moorhouse?) - 3:30"

"Peter Duncan did something around 3hrs 10mins I seem to remember. I was shocked as my only marathon attempt at that time was 4hrs 38mins. I always thought he was a tosser up to that point."

"Sorry but can someone explain why being big is a disadvantage...surely long legs go faster? Peter Duncan blimey. Perhaps he got a taxi round part of the course?"

"I said that it was a shame he had to pull out with injury and I'm sure that regardless of anything else the man must have a real competitive spirit (he's an Olympic gold medallist for Christ's sake) and must be really annoyed at not being able to give it a go. I hope he gives it another go, and I'll be fascinated to see how he does (as long as he doesn't beat my PB!)"

15. London to Brighton 2008

Running not cycling

Following a marathon PB in London that April, and an Ironman PB in Austria in July it was time to reward myself with "something completely different". An Ironman friend, Jonesy, was coming up with weird and wonderful races I had never heard of.

This one was no exception, and by coincidence, would begin in Greenwich Park where the start of the London Marathon is. The race was London to Brighton with a twist, cross-country! Like all of these types of races there are a handful of dedicated volunteers, highly enthusiastic race organisers and a small band of runners mad enough to be taking part.

Typically, there would be 200 or so runners and I have no idea how they would make any money - they must do it for the love of coming up with crazy races. The idea is straight forward, start at Blackheath and end up somewhere at the race finish (small tent and a race banner) in the middle of Brighton. The distance is fifty-eight miles, but this won't be down the A23 and a right turn at Croydon, this was to be all cross-country.

A letter arrived in late August to outline the details and rules of the race together with a 28-page A5 map book. This wasn't an off-the shelf map book. It had been painstakingly put together by the race organisers and they must have created 200 of them or so. Each page had a section of an ordnance survey map printed on the left-hand side of the page and some basic typed instructions alongside it like "At the bottom of the high street go past the railway station, then the police station. Take the left fork onto the road and look for the correct turning to the right and from there, the footpath next to the school".

You can probably imagine how the race broke down into small groups with some frantically trying to read the instructions and others waiting to be told which way to run.

Having re-found the map in my memorabilia box each page is covered in my handwriting which I had added during the race briefing. Comments like "Keston Common – Take Care" "Sharp right into driveway, through gate, left through high hedge, between two gardens" "Dry Hill Farm", "Beeches Farm" "Great Water Farm" "Wallhill Farm" "Burnthouse Farm" "Goat Farm – Go to right of farm buildings, follow path, left fork to woods" – I think you get the picture.

I tried to find out if the race is still being run. There seems to be a new one called London to Brighton 100k which began in 2012. It starts in Richmond-upon-Thames and makes its way to Brighton via the North and South downs. It looks like the original Trailwalker event but with 2,000 runners. Here are the top line instructions for the original 2008 race.

Dear Runner

Please find enclosed the running map book for the London to Brighton 2008. Please note the Ordnance Survey map references at the back of it. You may edit or annotate the map as you wish and supplement it or replace it with your own maps as you see fit. You are not allowed by the rules of this event, however, to upload the map to a GPS system for use on the day. You may rehearse parts of the route if you wish. There will be further hints and assistance given on the day at the briefing (06:30 at the start line). Please have a pen or pencil available to mark the map on the morning of the event. Your running number is written at the bottom of the page. The run will start at 07.00 sharp by General Wolfe's statue in Greenwich Park, London SE10. Registration will be just outside the main (top) gates to Blackheath as marked on the map from about 05:30. On the day you are responsible for bringing the map book, a pen or pencil, drinks bottles, favourite drinks, electrolytes, suitable clothing, food and/or gels, a compass, 4 safety pins, a mobile phone, cash for emergencies, and a bag for the clothing you wish us to transfer to the finish. If you need to drop out of the event on the day, please endeavour to find you way to the nearest checkpoint. There is an emergency number to telephone on the day of the event if you are injured, need to withdraw, or are genuinely completely lost (this is on the foot of each page of your map book). If you are lost, we will try to assist you but if we offer practical help in the form of transport you will be disqualified from the event. You have 12 hours to complete the event and you must reach the checkpoints at the times set out on the course part of the website or you will not be able to complete it (stage 2 after 3:55, stage 3 after 5:40, stage 4 after 8 hours and stage 5 after 9:45 arriving in Brighton by 1900 hours). We reserve the right to withdraw struggling competitors at our discretion for your safety. We promise our best efforts for a safe and enjoyable race for all, and we wish you all the very best on the day.

Yours faithfully, Extreme Running Limited

The start of the race was through the streets of Greenwich. One guy, from New Zealand I think, moved off fast and I later discovered he had already reccied the course a couple of weeks earlier, so he was soon out of sight. Small groups of the rest of us struggled with reading and running at the same time.

Periodically, there was a realisation that we had gone the wrong way and some back tracking before getting back on course. I was struggling with map reading so each time we stopped as a group I got my map out, looked meaningfully at it, and waited till someone seemed to know what they were doing and where we should be going.

As the race got outside of London and into the Sussex countryside the map reading got harder and harder as we trudged along smaller trails and across more farms and fields and through wooded paths.

Ironman Jonesy and another running mate of his were more cyclists and swimmers than runners, and after about four of five hours I was off with a group of three at the front of the race but behind the Kiwi guy. I was freeloading a lot on the map reading I must admit and by about 6 or 7 hours in I was purely focussed on running between whatever point on the map we were at and where we had to go next.

We were keeping a pretty good time as this is a 58-mile race. Coming up to 8 hours or so, the infamous Ditchling Beacon came into view and at that point I could pretty much work my way into Brighton blindfold having cycled it a few times. We went up the trail side of the hill and as we emerged at the top, we stuck together for a while before the run down to the finish and I came in second in a time of 8:40.

As a completely unselfish runner, I decided not to wait for Ironman Jonesy, as I had no idea where he was on the course, and I got the next train back to London and was back home in Chiswick for a few glasses of Rose with my wife by about 8PM.

The phone rang, Jonesy had bailed out of the race having got lost and ran out of time and daylight. He was sitting in a pub somewhere along the course waiting for race control to pick him up.

These types of races, where times don't matter, count towards the building and maintenance of a 'Sub-3 ready' level of fitness. 2008 turned out to be my peak performance year and races like this made it so enjoyable and privileged to have had the opportunity to run it. Thank you Extreme Running Limited!

16. Town to Tring 2009
The Canal Turn

Following on from the bonkers London to Brighton race a few months earlier, me and Ironman Jonesy were keen to seek out more barbaric blood-blistering races to break up the monotony of regular Ironman and marathon races. He discovered one called Town to Tring, and back, which seemed to fit the bill perfectly except I had a company Christmas party to attend on the Saturday evening of the race.

There were two parts to it: Part 1 run from London to Tring, Part 2 run from Tring to London. Distance forty-four miles each way along the Grand Union Canal from Brentford avoiding any wrong turns and not ending up in Oxford somewhere instead of Tring.

Like London to Brighton, we were soon sent an A5 race guidebook and told to assemble at the Premier Inn in Brentford on race day morning, in the middle of January. Lots of runners would make the big mistake of wearing layers and carrying rain jackets.

For me, lots of layers was a big no-no, no matter what the time of year. My circulation isn't that great but the fact you are running will keep you warm and within a few miles I knew I would regret any extra weight, so better off starting with as little as possible, including nutrition.

This race was during my peak weight, pace and fitness period based on all the ongoing Ironman training and newfound Sub-2.50 marathon times. Although this is a 44-mile race and times don't matter, I was in the mood to go out front and go fast. If it's along a canal then it's going to be flat, just a few lumps and bumps up and down locks. I was hoping for a Sub-5 or faster, which would effectively be Sub-3 pace but for a marathon and a half on top.

Within a mile or two a few likely lads had taken up pole position and it became clear that one of the five of us would win this. We meandered along quiet misty canal paths, around lock-gates, up and over various obstacles before five became three and eventually just me and another fella who seemed to be keen on a trophy.

You instinctively know when you are feeling good and you have gears left and when you don't, and this was one of those good days for me. I upped the pace with about fifteen miles or so to go and after a while it was just me, the canal, and people on house boats waking up and making breakfast.

These races are not set up like a major marathon with marshals and barriers to keep you on the course. You must rely on faded signposts and arrows here and there or you can end up miles off course in the middle of nowhere. At least the canal was a big clue, but there are no signs like 'Tring 2 miles' or anything.

So, I almost missed the "take the small stairs round the left-hand bend just before Tring" instruction and having emerged from the top of the stairs, onto a quiet country road there was no clue which way the country park hotel was where the race would finish. I flagged an oncoming taxi down and asked for directions to the hotel, (no I didn't get in it) and about ten minutes later arrived, victorious where a couple of people were setting up a table to check us in.

A decent time of 4:40 and the second guy turned up about ten minutes later. I thought I had won but was reminded by the organisers that you must run back the following day and win with a combined time.

I had the dilemma of a company Christmas party that night back in London, but I vowed to return to Tring the following morning. After the inevitable heavy night of drinking, I woke to the sound of my alarm, turned the alarm off, went back to sleep, and left second guy and the rest of them to it.

I think he was the overall winner as the challenge was there and back, not just there. There are dozens of these bonkers races if you search them out and they are great for building base fitness and not getting bored pounding the same old streets and races over and over again.

17. Endurance Life Trails 2010-17
A new addiction

Having finished the London 2010 Marathon just seven seconds the right side of my ninth Sub-3 then maybe things were getting tighter as I was getting older and maybe I needed something new. A very fast friend (Kona Ironman qualifier) asked if I fancied some off-road marathons. No chance of a Sub-3 on these things he said, but great training without the pressure of a time deadline. Seemed to make sense.

I had never heard of Endurance Life before, but their website showed a series of coastal path marathons running from September to May and the final race of the season was in Exmoor and was still open to entry. My very fast mate (Kona Jonesy, brother of IM Jonesy) had signed up already so why not. A few weeks later and I am walking down a steep hill from the field car park to a pub at the bottom and the race HQ where I met up with Kona Jonesy. He had camped overnight and looking around it felt like Glastonbury but for a running festival.

There were three distances, 5k, 10k and Marathon and of the 500 hundred or so people signing up, about 100 were going for the marathon. I had noticed the website listed each race on a scale of 1-5 with 5 being the most extreme. The grading was based on the amount of climb on the course and the steepness of certain sections as well as runs across beaches and the odd river here and there.

Exmoor was listed as a grade 5, the only such grade in the series, but surely that's just a few hills and a scenic run across a handful of cliff tops. Mandatory equipment included a phone, a whistle, headgear, bottles for water, a first aid kit and a foil blanket which was checked before the start. For those of us going for a serious time this could be minimised to keep the weight down by trying to pass off two plasters and some Nurofen as a 'first aid kit'.

The pre-race briefing detailed the need to look out for and follow small red arrows along the route (not to blindly follow the person in front as I was planning to do) and that the course was closer to 27 or 28 miles but that meant we were getting better value for money which was par for the course on these races. So far so good.

Staying with Kona Jonesy should get me a podium finish and the first mile or so was straight forward along a flat path through a wooded glade. Maybe I can win this? Shortly after, a red arrow directed us left and the start of the first steep hill began. Twenty of us dropped to fifteen, then to ten, and I watched helplessly as the front group disappeared out of sight and I realised I was in trouble less than two miles in.

This was a completely different game. This was not a metronomic 6:30 pace to be held mile in mile out that can be transferred from one race in one country to another, this is a series of one-off courses, and every turn delivers a knee shattering downhill or a heart-breaking climb with an occasional flat section for a moment or two of normality and sanity. Tree roots, rocks and man-made steps are trip traps that will bring you down like a sack of spuds if you don't focus constantly on what's beneath you. In a road race you look forwards, in a trail race you look downwards!

By the halfway point, if you even knew where the halfway point was, this was beginning to hurt, and hurt bad. A podium target started to give way to a finish target, then to a survival target. Time and pace were no longer a concern. Staying on course and not missing checkpoints and arrows and crosses becomes paramount. Go wrong and you could add another two miles to the course just to find your way back to where you went wrong.

I would never run with any sort of fancy GPS watch, just a basic Timex Casio. No mileage beeps, no distance splits, no stopwatch. It's all too distracting, you simply need to run the pace your body can handle and learn to understand it. All you really need to know is the time you started and what the time is now.

For a road marathon I would check the first mile pace then 5k, then 10k, then half-way, then focus on my mind and body and whether I was staying with those around me or dropping back. If your mind or body starts to slip, then hang in and hold on or let go.

A trail race has no mile markers and there is no knowledge of the hills and drops to come (for those like me who didn't pay attention at the pre-race briefing at least). You simply don't know how far in you are, how far there is to go, and what surprises await.

For the Exmoor run, we eventually emerged into a town call Lynton or Lynmouth, not sure which, and we were now running on flat roads and streets. We were probably three or four hours into the race, and I was well beyond the 'I'm done with this' stage, but surely now this was a run to the finish, and we are on familiar road terrain, right up my street. I could see a couple of runners ahead of me and it would only be a matter of time before they were hunted down and passed. Advantage me. About a hundred yards later, and gaining fast, the runners ahead suddenly disappeared out of sight.

Thankfully, I could see one of the small red arrow signs signalling left, so I followed the instruction and ended up at what looked like a train station with one single old-fashioned train carriage. Rising above the station was an almost vertical railway track going straight up as far as the eye could see through a cutting in the trees.

There must be some mistake, maybe someone turned the arrow round, surely, they didn't expect us to have to run up a vertical incline on an old railway track. Did they?

Having done zero course reconnaissance prior to the race, I was completely unaware of what I later discovered is the fully operational Lynton & Lynmouth Cliff railway built in 1888 and is billed as the world's highest and steepest fully water powered railway. Rising 500 feet at a gradient of 58% all we must do is run up it.

Luckily, for us 'runners' at least, someone had built a walkway that zig zagged the railway from left to right, so no need to catch the actual train but just get on and walk it, climb it, crawl it or whatever it would take to get this nightmare over with.

At the top I was pretty much at my wits end with this type of racing and having caught up with a runner resting on a gate before the next section, I asked if he had any idea how far the finish was. He had a Garmin of some kind so was able to guess we still had four, five, or even six, miles to go.

I just wanted to lay down and cry. I walked, jogged, and staggered my way to the finish in a disrespectful time of 5:01:52, over 2 hours slower than the London Marathon a few weeks earlier. In cycling terms this is mountain biking vs road racing, both on bikes, but that's where the similarity ends. Having paced with the front runners at the start I had slipped to 23rd place out of 186 finishers.

Kona Jonesy was already back and relaxing with a beer and a burger, having nailed it in 03:44:41 and finishing in 1st place. Serious respect. Having parted company with Kona Jonesy to drive back to London, stating never to run one of these things ever again, I signed up for their full ten race package running from September later that year through to May 2011.

The Isle of Wight, Dorset, Gower, Portland, Anglesey, South Devon, Pembrokeshire, Sussex, and Flete. Sadly (thankfully) Exmoor clashed with the London Marathon date, so I never got a chance to return.

Within this 10-month period I was to cram in four road marathons (Dublin, Tokyo, Mablethorpe, and London) and two Ironman marathons assuming no Ironman DNF's before or during the run.

Over a ten-year period, I returned twenty-six times to run and re-run Endurance Life Marathons and Ultra's with a podium finish in five. I didn't keep an ongoing record of my times as times were not important as each race terrain is totally different with different levels of extremity, but I contacted Endurance Life to recover them all. Not that time's matter here but the average time across all twenty-six races I ran was 4:43:59.

For those of you who haven't considered this type of running it's a perfect way of building your base fitness and maintaining it due to the frequency of events between September and May. It gets you through the winter months with races to book and look forward to. They are all in the UK and are in some of the most beautiful parts of the country wherever there is a National Trust Trail.

There are a variety of distances all happening on the same day, so you can take friends, partners and even pets (dogs) to do different distances. You will visit places you otherwise wouldn't, and surprise yourself with how beautiful this country is.

For example, I had never been to Northumberland before, and this is a race of 26 miles from one castle to another. It's not a loop race so you get to run 26 miles up the Northumberland coastline along beaches and hills and cliffs, expecting a Viking invasion to land to your right at any moment.

You are adding to the local coastal economy vs big cities and in-land destinations who probably don't need it as much. You will get to meet a whole new type of runner and running comrades. I can't recommend it strongly enough. In case you're interested here is my full Endurance Life races record from 2010 to 2017.

YEAR	MNTH	RACE	DISTANCE	TIME	PODIUM
2010	MAY	EXMOOR	MARA	05:01:52	
2010	SEP	ISLE OF WIGHT	MARA	04:11:40	
2010	OCT	DORSET	MARA	04:41:41	
2010	NOV	GOWER	MARA	04:28:47	
2010	DEC	PORTLAND	MARA	03:59:28	
2011	JAN	ANGLESEY	MARA	04:07:16	
2011	FEB	SOUTH DEVON	MARA	04:34:55	
2011	MAR	SUSSEX	MARA	04:29:07	
2011	MAR	PEMBROOK	MARA	03:53:54	BRONZE
2011	MAY	FLETE	MARA	04:29:17	
2011	OCT	NORTHUMBERLAND	MARA	03:37:12	GOLD
2011	DEC	GOWER	ULTRA	06:07:39	GOLD
2012	JAN	ANGLESEY	ULTRA	07:08:30	
2012	FEB	PORTLAND	MARA	04:17:35	SILVER
2012	MAR	SUSSEX	MARA	04:09:30	
2012	MAY	FLETE	MARA	05:15:16	
2012	OCT	PEMBROOK	MARA	04:26:11	SILVER
2012	NOV	GOWER	MARA	05:04:52	
2012	DEC	DORSET	ULTRA	06:10:27	
2013	FEB	SOUTH DEVON	MARA	05:24:52	
2013	MAY	NORTH YORK MOORS	MARA	04:03:54	
2014	FEB	NORTHUMBERLAND	MARA	03:58:38	
2015	NOV	GOWER	MARA	05:29:21	
2016	FEB	NORTHUMBERLAND	MARA	04:14:22	
2017	FEB	NORTHUMBERLAND	MARA	04:38:30	
2017	MAR	SUSSEX	MARA	05:12:22	

18. Dublin Marathon 2010
The S3XX Tattoo

Arriving home from the Dublin 2010 marathon, and by now ten Sub-3's in the bag, I was noticing a distinct lack of interest from my two sons who were now in their early and mid-teens.

To them it was just another race of many and for me, approaching fifty, was it time to retire from this quest which was beginning to lose its purpose both for me and evidently those close to me.

Having just signed up for a series of ten Endurance Life coastal path marathons, where no-one would Sub-3, then maybe that was the perfect excuse to enjoy the run and the scenery and forget the time.

But London, in particular, has a hold on anyone who can still qualify under their Good for Age times. Each qualifying time entitles you to run the following two years of the race.

Given how hard it is to get in on the ballot, this was a running treadmill that was hard to get off. Better to fall off one day, when the times are no longer there, than to get off prematurely with race slots in the bank. If you can do ten Sub-3's then why not twenty?

Certainly, twenty sounded better than ten and with eleven Ironman races completed there was a new target here somewhere. I enrolled myself into the newly formed

20-20 club which to my knowledge no-one was yet a member. The entry fee for members would be 20 Sub-3's and 20 Ironman's. So, just 10 more of each to go, but at the age of fifty maybe not a lot of time left to do it. To keep my sons interested, I announced they would get a free trip to Las Vegas as soon as I had completed 20 Sub-3's (they would probably be old enough to drink in the USA by then).

And what about a tattoo to go alongside the IM one? S3XX – that's the boy! We're no longer chasing a time; we're now chasing a tatt.

There must be a purpose to this stuff. It can't just be banging it out race after race. I'm getting older by the day and sooner or later my body will give up even if my mind doesn't.

Since I started writing this memoir, I have been seeking out Sub-3 runners and multiple Sub-3 runners. I have found quite a few but I have yet to meet anyone who has Sub-3'd twenty times or more in officially recorded race times.

Even professional marathon runners would struggle to do this as the sheer intensity of race training for them at that level takes a massive toll on their body. To run world record paces can't be done week in and week out and inevitably injury causes them to pull out of major races and forces them to focus on selected races maybe once or twice per year at most.

19. Boston Marathon 2012
The Big Daddy

The Boston Marathon is different. In my opinion, it is the most prestigious of all marathons. A Sub-3 Boston is a level up from a standard Sub-3 and qualifying for this race is very special. The race is run every year in April on Patriots' Day which is a Monday, and it is typically six days before the London Marathon. I entered for the 2012 race by accident.

I simply forgot to register for London 2012. I had already secured a Good for Age slot and received the confirmation e-mail, but I forgot to complete the registration by the deadline and didn't realise. I called the race office, pleaded, and blamed them for losing my application, but they said 'no'.

This would be a first London marathon miss in years and to have given up a guaranteed slot was unforgiveable given how hard it is to get in. I would simply have to register again in 2013.

So now what? What other marathons are there in April? Wait a minute, Boston! Surely that was closed for entry. But no, there was still time to register by a few weeks.

Boston is 95% qualification runners and the qualification times by age and sex are tough. They give you a window of proven times up until 18 months before the race, so my 2:52 Dublin time was easily strong enough. But unlike other marathon qualification times, there is a twist. They announce the time you must meet by sex and age-group. When registration open's they start the process with those that have gone twenty minutes better than their qualifying time, then move to ten minutes, then five minutes and so on. Imagine you had to hit 3 hours to qualify, only to find out that you had to be 10 minutes better than that to get in.

There is an 89% chance of qualifying, even if you have first achieved the qualifying time, which means about 3,000 runners each year who qualify, fail to get a place because of the number of registrations that beat the qualifying time. The 2017 breakdown of qualifiers by qualifying time is below.

- 4,357 Qualifiers met their qualifying time by 20 minutes or faster.
- 7,105 Qualifiers met their qualifying time by 10 minutes or faster.
- 6,845 Qualifiers met their qualifying time by 05 minutes or faster.
- 4,497 Qualifiers met their qualifying time by 02 minutes or faster.

Having researched what this means in practice vs qualifying for other marathons I came across this comparison of the Boston Marathon with the New York Marathon.

"The average New York Marathon finish times for women aged 18-34 for example, was 4 hours 36 minutes. The qualifying time for the Boston Marathon the same year for women aged 18-34 was 3 hours 35 minutes. In essence, if a female (age 18-34) wants to run the Boston Marathon, she must run a marathon one hour faster than the average New York Marathon finish time to qualify."

The race has four starts coloured Red, White, Blue, and Yellow with eight Pens of 8,000 people starting each stage or wave. Red wave qualifying is mostly Sub-3 or below, White below 3:30, Blue below 3:56 and Yellow for the rest. Age doesn't matter only your qualifying time counts in terms of wave and pen allocation. To make Pen 1 of the Red Start is at least a Sub-2:45 qualify.

You truly feel that you are surrounded by serious runners, no rhino costumes, no superheroes, no people running as different types of fruit and vegetables or in wedding dresses and deep-sea diver outfits, this is the real deal.

I qualified in Red Wave Pen 3, which is success in and of itself, and if any running number is worth keeping afterwards, it's that one. When the gun goes off it's as though all eight Pens are up and running at race pace within less than fifty yards, like a Formula 1 Start grid where all cars are away at the same time with no queue or crush unlike other marathons. It really is special.

Arriving in Boston for 2012, I boarded the underground tram from the airport and kept myself to myself. Other runner types were clearly on the train. I overhead a very loud conversation between some Boston Celtic basketball fans and some bewildered runners "Are you running the race on Monday?" "Yeah" "Man you are going to die out there?" My ears pricked up. "They say, it's going to be 90 degrees even at the start and climbing from there". Oh no! I hadn't checked the weather.

It's April for god's sake! I also only had jeans and heavy T-Shirts with me. Heat is my nemesis. I am a reptile at heart and must stay cool, always. The slightest increase in temperature and my body starts to sweat. Warm drinks at aid stations might as well be a cup of sick and I always drink my wine with lots of ice cubes. Callipo lollies and ice-cold smoothies from Starbucks or Costa are sought out quickly after every race.

So, a complete train wreck situation begins to unfold. I landed quite late in the evening and although it felt warm there was nothing to worry about until the Boston Celtic fans put the cat firmly among the pigeons. The following day was boiling hot from sunrise to sunset, without a cloud in the sky from dawn to dusk. First job, buy some shorts and lighter shirts, second job register for the race, third job back to the hotel to cool down and pray for an overnight rainstorm. Fat chance.

Early race day morning and the hot sun was already rising. This is not an early morning start like most marathons. It's a 10am start and by the time I reached the start area people were finding whatever shade they could. With minutes to go to the start gun and with the National Anthem being played, I was still sitting outside Pen 3 on the Red Start under the porch of a nearby house.

With 30 seconds to go I left the porch; joined the pen and we set off into what felt like a blazing inferno. It's a point-to-point race and appears to be downhill for the first half, which is deceiving as it's undulating ups and downs along the way make it hard to set a consistent pace.

As advertised, Wellesley Girls College can be heard from a mile away as you approach the half-way mark, where screaming college students make you feel they turned out just to cheer you on and this gives you a momentary lift of hope that your race is still on track. Heartbreak Hill does what it says on the tin at Mile 20, and whatever hope you may have had left of going Sub-3 is taken from you on that two-kilometre incline.

The temperature that day peaked at 89f (32c). Almost, 4,000 people, and many of the elite athletes, pulled out before the start of the race based on the promise of a guaranteed slot the following year. More than 2,000 were treated on the course during the race, and 120 were treated in hospital.

For me the Sub-3 dream became a Sub-4 target soon into the race and after dipping in under 3:50, I made my way back round to the finish line via the medical tent for a life-saving mango smoothie from the Starbucks directly next to the finish line.

This would be the same spot where one of two bombs would go off the following year killing three and injuring two-hundred-and-eighty spectators and runners. This would also be part of a 2013 schedule to run all the six marathon majors in the same year.

In case you are thinking of running the Boston Marathon then typical corral times and sizes are shown below. Within each wave are eight corrals or pens.

Bib numbers 101 through 7,700 have run qualifying times faster than 3:07:27 and are in the Red wave, which starts at 10:02 a.m.

Bib numbers 8,000 through 15,600 have run qualifying times between 3:07:27 and 3:27:17 and are in the White wave, which starts at 10:25 a.m.

Bib numbers 16,000 through 23,600 have run qualifying times between 3:27:17 and 3:56:54 and are in the Blue wave, which starts at 10:50 a.m.

Bib numbers 24,000 through 32,500 have run qualifying times greater than 3:56:54 and are in the Yellow wave, which starts at 11:15 a.m.

The Boston Marathon and The London Marathon both announced within days of each other that they will introduce a non-binary entry and qualifying category for 2023 race schedules. As of 2023 this now applies to all World Majors except for the Tokyo marathon who have yet to follow suit

London has announced that this only applies to the mass start racers, so presumably the ballot and charity places where there is no condition for a qualifying time anyway. For Professional, Elite and Good for Age, qualifiers then biological male and biological female qualification categories are maintained. So, it seems like you can be non-binary unless you want to qualify for a guaranteed slot based on proof of time.

Boston, which is, more-or-less a 100% qualification race, have stated that people who identify as non-binary can qualify on the biological female qualification time categories. That would seem to enable biological men two ways of qualifying for Boston, one within the biological men's qualifying levels and the other within the biological female category if they identify as non-binary.

The biological female qualification categories are about thirty minutes slower than that for biological men. It's not clear if they will publish and record three categories of results or whether non-binary results will be wrapped into the biological men or biological women's result categories.

It will be interesting to see how this ruling will work out when all of the 2023 races are run and how it impacts the results. It's difficult to have an opinion either way until the impact on biological women and men's qualification slots are known. In the London Marathon 2023, 88 people ran as non-binary and three finished Sub-3.

As far as the quest for a Sub-3 goes, nothing changes. Whatever your sex or gender, Sub-3 is Sub-3. The clock waits for no-one.

20. Tokyo Marathon 2013

A new World Major

Working for a Japanese corporation headquartered in Tokyo has some advantages. In 2011 I managed to get one of the senior executives to help me enter the Tokyo Marathon and promptly created a business trip there to coincide. The general chaos of Tokyo to an English-speaking foreigner and the labyrinth of trains and taxis needed to get to the start on time was a challenge.

For the 2011 race, I committed a schoolboy error that occurred during the race which you might want to note as it applies to most marathons except for those in the UK and USA. Having worked my way from about Pen 5 to Pen 1 to get to the front of the start and not risk being held hostage by slower runners in the first part of the race, I found myself well inside the first 100 runners or so as we took off down through the start area and onto the city streets.

Tokyo is a fast marathon, especially as the front third or so of the race is a gradual decline down towards Tokyo Bay. But this was feeling really fast, and I was eagerly awaiting the first mile marker to get a fix on how quick, or slow, I was running.

I'm not one for wearing a Garmin watch or any other fancy GPS device and I don't always use the stopwatch function on my somewhat basic Ironman Timex, but it can help for the first mile or two if there are no official clocks on the course at every mile marker. London for example doesn't have an official race clock until the Mile-3 marker, when the runners from different starts, merge together.

As we approached and passed the first mile marker I glanced down at my stopwatch, and it said something like 4:05. Clearly there was something wrong as I was expecting between 6:00 and 6:30 so I chose to ignore the watch and run to the beat of my body.

As we approached the second mile marker I glanced down again, and it said something like 8:10. Something wrong here. At this point it stated to dawn on me that these were kilometres and not miles.

It hadn't crossed my mind that we were running metric, not imperial, and this is a 42k race not a 26.2m. I frantically started to work out what on earth my KM pace needed to be but dividing three hours by forty-two kilometres without a calculator was going to be tricky.

I eventually thought to break it down to 10k's and figured out that 4 X Sub 40 10k's would be 160 minutes leaving 20 minutes to do the final 2k and that felt about right. If 10k is forty minutes, then 5k needs to be twenty minutes or thereabouts and from then on, I simply got a check on every 5k and 10k until about 30k when you might as well switch off from thinking about the clock and run to your body. It did work though and for metric marathons afterwards that was the general checkpoint I would follow.

For Tokyo 2011, everything worked out fine and with another Sub-3 in the bags towards the S3XX goal. In 2012, the pain of holding twenty-minute 5k's started to set in about the 30k mark and to my dismay the three-hour pacers passed me at around 35k.

I watched helplessly as they started to disappear up the road and on to the bridge before the run in to the finish. This was another Sub-3 that got away, and I finished in a disappointing 3:03:10.

For 2013, Tokyo was granted World Major Marathon status adding a new sixth major to the current five (Boston, London, Berlin, Chicago, and New York). This was a lucky coincidence for me as it set me up for the Big Six plan later that year (see Chapter 22).

There was a noticeable increase in the promotion and interest in the race under this new status and for me the 2013 race started the year on a high with a comfortable Tokyo PB of 2:56:41 which made it S3XIV in the quest for S3XX.

At the age of 52 I was clearly still able to knock out a decent pace and all doubts from the previous year's failed attempt were now forgotten and faith was fully restored.

Now that Tokyo had been elevated to this new status, runners everywhere were adding it to their bucket list of marathon races that had to be run.

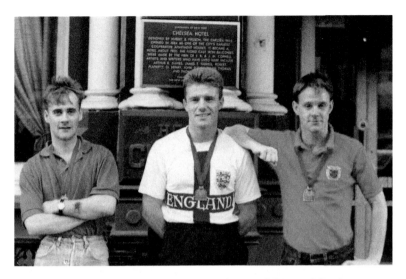

1990 NYC Marathon – The Start of Something!

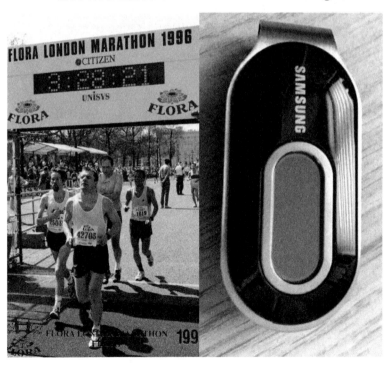

London 1996 – Not even close   **Sub-3 Soundtrack**

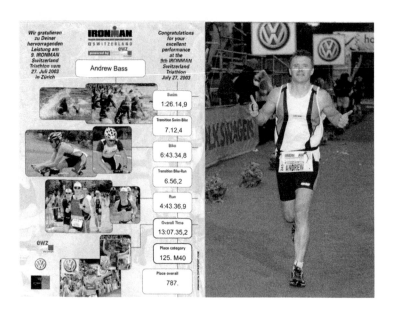

2003 – Wild Horses and a different type of marathon

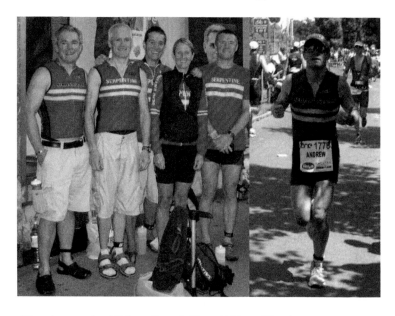

The Jonesy's, Rhino Guy & Fast Wife – The Ironman Years

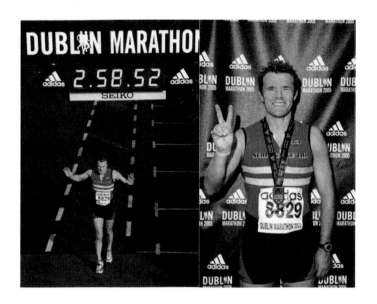

2005 Fifteen years in the making – V for Victory and '2'

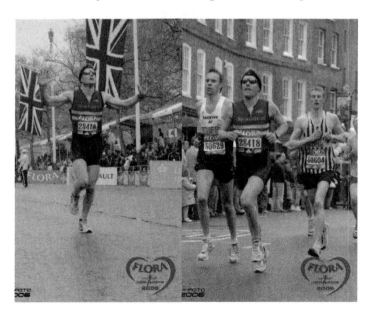

2006 London – In fast company

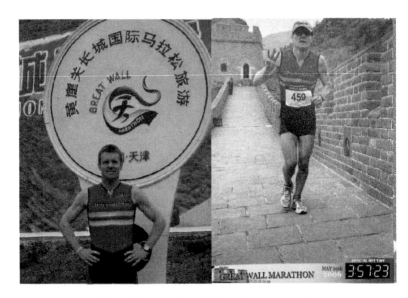

2006 - Hitting The Wall – The Great One

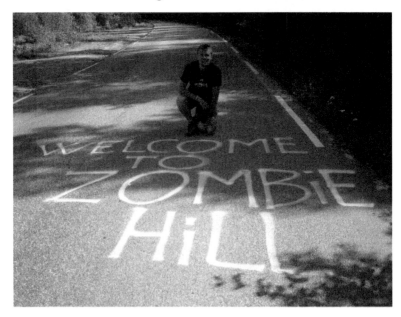

2006 – A Norseman Black and Zombie Hill

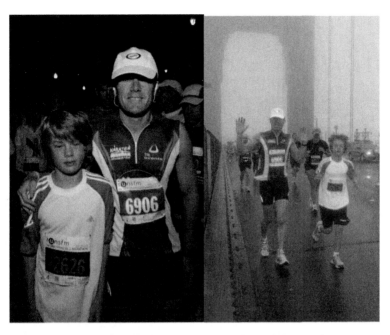

2007 – Sons of San Francisco - The Golden Gate

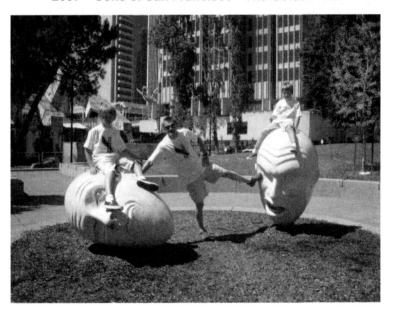

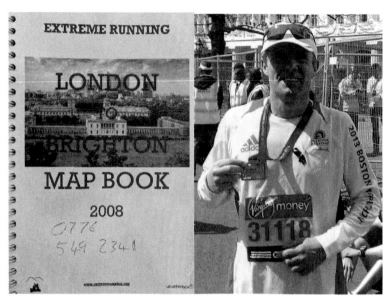

2008/9 Going very long　　　**2013 – Big Six double-header**

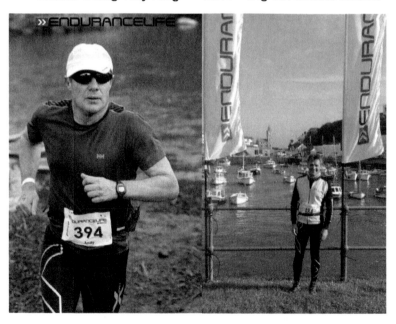

2010-17 Endurance Life coastal path marathons

110

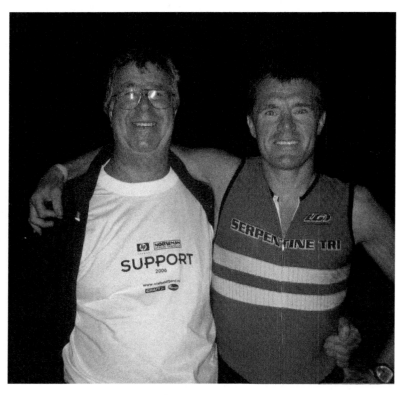

Race day and week support crew

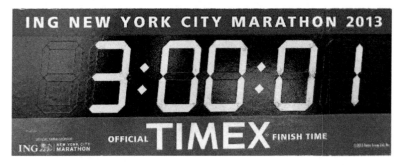

A timely reminder on the fridge of how not to do it!

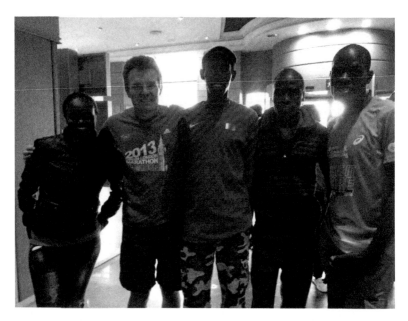

2015 Barcelona Marathon & Sub-3 Podium Gods

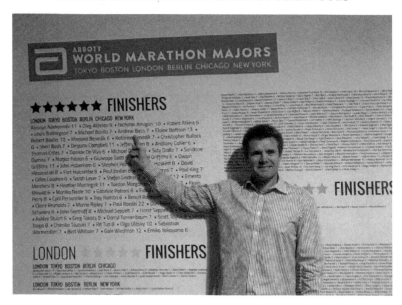

2015 London Marathon & the first listing of 6* finishers

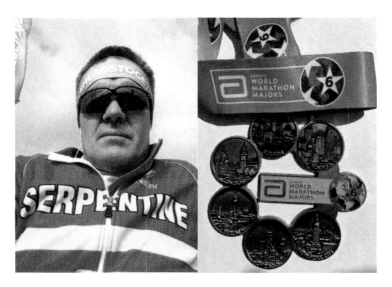

2017 – The end of something and something to show for it

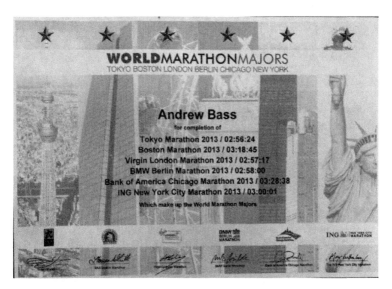

Dear Guinness – A World 1st – Where is my official record?

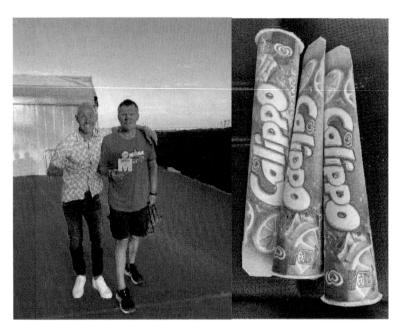

2022 – Kona Guy (another podium) and top nutrition

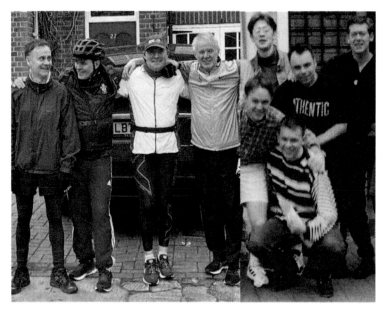

2023 – The 1990 crew – one last time – RIP Bren

21. Boston Marathon 2013

The year of the bomb

Having tasted Boston, the previous year this was now priority over London, given they are within six days of each other. I had entered both of them and the target was to Sub-3 both.

The plan was to finish Boston and get on a recovery drip at the medical tent in the finish area, I had spent an hour there recovering on a bed after the 2012 race, that had been 90 degrees heat all day and thousands of runners had either pulled out at the start, collapsed along the course, or ended up in the medical tent at the end.

From there, the plan was to get a mango smoothie at Starbucks near the finish line as I had done in 2012. Then off to the airport and catch the 6-7pm flight out of Boston to Heathrow that night. From there, prepare for the London Marathon six days later the following Sunday. I changed the hotel choice from 2012 to be near to the finish rather than near to the start and to get a quick shower at the hotel afterwards and off to the airport in time for tea and medals.

Delta Air out 09.40 from Heathrow to land 12.30 Saturday and get the local transport to the Aquarium Tube Station directly opposite The Harborside Inn in Downtown Boston. Check-In and straight out to the Registration Centre on Boylston Street with a good chance to soak in the atmosphere and watch everything being set up for the race on Monday. A bit of R&R

Sunday and a chance to have a Guinness, or two, in the Boston pubs which all seemed to be full of people celebrating being Irish for the weekend (thought that was in March!).

Race day was smoother than expected as the buses taking people out to the start at Hopkinton were regular and taking Red start runners first so no stress so far. Although it meant getting up a bit earlier than staying near to Hopkinton the previous year, the plan for the Boston-London Sub-3 double-header was starting well.

The temperature was cool compared to the previous year and, arriving an hour and a half before the start, I laid on the grass and slept a while. The euphoria of qualifying to run this event and being here and mingling with serious runner types was starting to set in. I have covered everything about qualifying and the race history earlier, so I won't go over it again.

The cooler temperature meant taking in more of the atmosphere at the start and enjoying it vs the previous year of the heatwave and the mad panic for shade and water and anywhere to get out of the sun. If your goal is to go Sub-3 then it doesn't matter where or when you do it, but if you do manage to, then you should check whether it could get you a Boston qualifier place. If it does, then don't hesitate for a moment to do it.

This is a special race not just for marathon runners worldwide but for the whole city of Boston. It is run on Patriots Day weekend on the Monday and the whole city is out celebrating, with the marathon being the culmination of it. Having Sub-3'd Tokyo a few weeks earlier my confidence of a Sub-3 Boston was running reasonably high even though I now knew what the course was like and that it would require a lot in the split bank at halfway and that I would need to be feeling as if the race had only just started when I got there.

From memory in 2012, I knew the first half of the race was downhill but undulating and the second half would include Heartbreak Hill which, from memory, was steeper than expected.

The college girls at Wellesley were out making a real din and everyone seemed to up the pace in response despite the signs of pain beginning to appear in the eyes of those not wearing sunglasses. Approaching halfway I was not feeling great, but I had been holding a decent pace till then and I was pleasantly surprised to be at halfway in 1:26:43 which for any of the other five world major marathons would probably have meant a nailed-on Sub-3 barring a major incident.

But this is Boston, and that front half is deceivingly difficult in my opinion. I could feel my pace slowing long before Heartbreak Hill and I had given up checking times at each mile as the mental parrot on one shoulder was teasing the physical parrot on the other and they were in a battle as to which one would be giving out first. Once the parrot's move from positive to negative your Sub-3 race is over and halfway up Heartbreak Hill both parrots had won.

As soon as you walk, it's game over. You will talk yourself into it being just one quick walk and you can still do it but as the other runners start streaming past and giving you words of encouragement; your Sub-3 is gone. You will now start talking yourself into why a 3:05 would be respectable, then a 3:10, then thoughts of what the qualify time for next year is and so-on.

The Sub-3 back-to-back with London in six days' time was also disappearing as the hill got steeper and the walk got longer. I did manage to salvage some pace and pride as the sight of the city came into view and I managed to drag myself over the finish line in 3:18:45 (so a 1:27 1st half and a 1:51 2nd half if you are wondering how much deterioration can be), The run down the finish straight along Boylston Street was a real tear-jerking moment as the crowds are ten or twenty deep each side of the road.

The noise level is deafening and the finish gantry at the end of the street with all the Boston Police lined up is an incredible sight as you finish, and the reception you get from the volunteers is really special. I collected the famous Boston marathon medal, one of the good vs the bad and the ugly, and sauntered through the finish area of food, drink, and finishers shirts.

The original plan had been to Sub-3 and go to the medical tent, fake illness, and get a drip in my arm to set me up for London six days later. But with a 3:18 this plan was in tatters, so I decided to move on, get a Mango Frap from Starbucks back at the finish line, as I had done the previous year.

I had an hour or two to kill before getting my bag and a shower at the hotel and off to the airport. I got to the intersection of where the runners are coming out of the race area and into the general crowd area where friends and family meet and go off together to celebrate.

I turned left onto Boylston Street to get to Starbucks, but the crowd was deep and hardly moving and I was also feeling a bit giddy and had an empty-sick moment (gagging air) by a fence.

I decided not to bother fighting my way back to the finish line area but instead turned back the other way and headed east along Boylston Street away from the finish line and proceeded back to the hotel across Boston Common listening to my Sub-3 soundtrack.

The race had started at 10am, I had taken three hours and eighteen minutes to run it so with twenty minutes or so messing around through the finish and a thirty-minute walk to the hotel this is probably just gone 2pm and my flight is taking off at 6.35pm so a few hours to kill.

The hotel wouldn't let me take a shower as I had checked out so I sat around the hotel lobby in my running kit and thought I would kill an hour there and then get moving. I figured I could get a shower at the airport if BA had one in their lounge, and I could blag my way in as a silver card holder even though I was travelling Delta Air.

The station for the train transit system was near the hotel and from memory I had to go a few stops east, change to another line and head out towards Logan International airport. As I was going down the stairs into the station a somewhat flustered station employee was running up the stairs in front of me and that's when I first heard about a problem.

"There may not be any trains down there sir, a bomb has gone off and they may close the station soon so you may need to find another route". He carried on past me clearly on a mission to get somewhere, "Sorry, did you say a bomb, what down there?" "No", he said, "over by the marathon".

I carried on down the stairs, as you do, and got to the platform just as a train arrived, which was pretty much empty, so I boarded it and headed off to the airport oblivious to the horrific scenes unfolding above ground.

There was no phone signal until I emerged at the airport to get a bus transfer to the terminal, and it was only then when I realised the dozens of texts appearing on the phone as clearly it was becoming headline news in the UK. Later people told me they felt I would be OK as the bomb had gone off about four hours and fifty minutes into the race and they had expected me to have finished the race by then.

A work colleague who had a close friend working at BA texted me to tell me that all flights in and out of Boston were being grounded, that the chances of getting out were slim and that I would probably be spending another night in Boston.

I carried on to the airport, still in running gear under a track suit, and the unfolding drama was clear to see as more and more FBI type agents and uniformed officers seemed to be arriving at the airport to check who was leaving the country in the early parts of the operation.

The queues at customs clearance started to build as everyone was being checked and double checked. Cancelled signs were beginning to appear on the scheduled outgoing flights and all incoming flights were being diverted to other airports.

Strangely the Delta flight to London still showed as On-Time with BA flights showing cancelled, so I was wandering around the airport waiting for the cancelled sign to appear, but it didn't.

It turned out that departures on flights that had already landed and were being turned around for departure, were being allowed out. Any flights that were coming in had been diverted so only a handful of flights including mine were OK to depart.

Boston ended up in a state of lockdown as the search for the bombers continued over four-and-a-half days until they eventually caught the remaining bomber hiding in a boat in someone's back yard. Had I not booked that flight out on Sunday, I would have ended up there for an unplanned extended stay.

As I boarded the plane there were two FBI agents making final checks – they seemed a bit surprised that someone who had run the marathon was already at the airport to fly out. They asked me what time I had finished, and I said 3:18 as the Sub-3 failure was still top of mind "After the bomb went off?" one of them asked, "No" I said, "I finished before it went off". They said the bomb went off before 3pm! I explained how I didn't know what time the bomb went off just my finish time. They let me on, the doors closed and after a couple of glasses of wine, I settled into an in-flight movie.

I never understood the full scale of it all until I was back in the UK the following day and reading about it in the newspapers and watching it on TV back home. It was shocking to watch and to discover that people had lost their lives and countless others were injured and many others seriously injured.

It changed marathon procedures straight after. London had initially questioned whether to go ahead and had introduced far more security bag checks at race day check-in.

The Chicago marathon limited the size of race-day check in bags and these were made as clear plastic so that all contents inside could be seen. At the New York Marathon all streets and roads around the finish area were shut off and the walk back after the marathon to the city centre seemed almost as long as the marathon itself.

The Boston marathon is special for all sorts of reasons and if you ever get the opportunity to run it then take it. There is, in my opinion, a special respect for running

Boston over and above that of any of the other World Marathon Majors.

At a recent wedding I got talking to someone who was an avid runner and had run a number of marathons, so we got down to comparing notes. She, being impressed with the quantity of marathons I had run, me being more impressed that she had Sub-3'd Boston a few years earlier in 2:56. Something I would never do.

To put it into perspective, 4,188 runners out of around 30,000 runners went Sub-3 in the Boston Marathon 2023. Only 3,034 runners out of around 50,000 runners went Sub-3 in the London Marathon 2023. Race conditions were similar.

On face value it appears that London is the harder course due to a lower percentage going Sub-3, but the reverse is true. Boston is simply the highest quality field in terms of race qualification requirements (See Chapter 26 – How the Big 6 differ).

Perhaps they should make some of those Top Trump Cards for marathon running, a Boston Sub-3 card would, in my opinion, be the Top Trump in the deck.

22. London Marathon 2013
The Big Six Plan

Hours after the Boston Marathon 2013 bomb on the Monday, the London Marathon scheduled in just 6 days' time was placed in doubt as the organisers grappled with the spectre of a similar thing happening and the fact that over 35,000 runners and their friends and families were making their way to the capital to run and watch the race.

Eventually, the decision was taken to run the race in solidarity with Boston. At 7am on the Tuesday before the race I found myself on the Piccadilly line from Heathrow reading the pages of coverage of what had happened just twelve hours or so earlier in Boston. Fellow passengers were looking across at my Boston 2013 race jacket and wondering if and how I could possibly have run that race less than a day earlier and be sitting on the same tube.

With the London Marathon race back on, several people at registration on Saturday, me included, were wearing Boston Marathon finisher shirts out of respect, solidarity, and some level of guilt. Like a handful of others, I wore the Boston finisher shirt for the race.

On the walk from Blackheath station to the starting pens, a guy sidled up to me and asked me about Boston and we got chatting. He soon announced he had run "all five" world majors over several years, and he seemed surprised I didn't know what that meant. He explained there are, or were, five World Marathon Majors, but from this year (2013) there are now six as Tokyo was made a major this year. "I haven't run Tokyo, but I've run the other five" he eagerly explained. "Oh ok" I said trying to sound interested. "What are the five?" I asked. "Well, six now he said so Tokyo, Boston, London, Berlin, Chicago and New York". "Oh ok, great" I replied, "I ran New York in 1990 so I guess I've done that one and I ran Tokyo this year, so I've done four of them I guess" We chatted for a while longer and parted as he went to the Blue pen, and I went to the Red one.

I went through the normal start rituals, queue for the loo, rest, queue for the loo, rest, queue for the loo one last time, Nurofen, Deep Heat, Endurance Life cap, shades, soundtrack, headphones, kit bag to truck, bin liner, start line, and relax.

Having failed miserably to add Boston to my growing list of Sub-3 conquests and this being just six days later and with jet lag and lactate probably still in my legs, but the potential of near perfect weather conditions, I was in two minds as to which way this might go.

Sure, I would, as always, pace a Sub-3 and hope to be well inside 1:30 at halfway. As normal, I would keep an eye on the clock at each mile marker to make sure the pace was high enough and, as always, I would revert to listening to my body for the second half of the race and ticking off each mile as being one closer to the finish. I crossed the halfway point in 1:25:22 so almost five minutes in hand.

The game now, as always was to hold each mile at that pace and hold that five minutes split advantage for as long as possible and then let adrenalin and confidence kick-in the closer to the latter miles we got. I had long since stopped worrying about the so called 'wall' at 18-19 miles, for me the 'wall' was a halfway thing. If you're in the 1:25 area and still feeling ok you are nailing it and you have some room for slippage in the second half, if it's in the 1:28-1:29 area then you are not leaving much room for the second half of the race so it's 50/50 from here on in.

The best 1st half I ever ran to go Sub-3 was London 2009 in 1:20:49 which delivered a 2:46:59 finish vs the 2008 Marathon where a 1:21:06 halfway delivered a 2:46:30 and an all-time PB. The worst half split time for a Sub-3 had been Dublin 2005 at 1:28:09.

Looking back on it, London 2013 wasn't memorable for the race itself in that it wasn't my first, my fastest, nor a particular milestone (Sub-3 number 15) but maybe under the circumstances of just six days after Boston it should have been more memorable than it had been at the time.

More importantly, had I not met the guy walking to the start at Blackheath who had planted the idea of running all six World Majors into my mind then I would have finished the race as normal and gotten on to planning more Ironman's, more Endurance Life races, and all sorts of other weird and wonderful races you can dig up if you want to.

Throughout the week my mind kept thinking about doing all six World Majors in say 2014. My latest London time would get me into any of them under a Good for Age qualify place.

I could easily wangle a business trip to Tokyo in February, it would be great to do Boston and London as a double header again in April so I would just need to plan for Berlin, Chicago, and New York whenever they were.

An hour or two of research later and I determined that Berlin was early October, Chicago late October and New York early November so the plan was coming together. 2014 would be the year of 'The Big Six'.

But something about the plan didn't feel right. Why wait until 2014 when you've already done the first three and it's still only April? Why not do the second three this year, who knows what may happen next year?

I only had Ironman Wales for September in the current race plan, plus several long-distance swim events. I had signed up for Endurance Life Marathons in May and October (between Chicago and New York) so this seemed doable.

To keep costs down, the USA races could be the normal fly on Friday, register and relax Saturday, race on Sunday, evening flight out, home for Monday.

But were these races already full and would I be able to get a Good for Age slot or an overseas runner slot or was it simply too late in the day?

The answer was 'no' and 'yes' across the board and by the end of that week all three races were entered, hotels and flights were booked and the second half of the Big Six was locked and loaded and that would mean all six in the same year.

Next stop, Berlin.

23. Berlin Marathon 2013
Russian Massage Guy

The Berlin 2013 Marathon was the 40th anniversary of the event and I had heard that Berlin was a fast course so this could be an ideal opportunity to add another Sub-3 to the list. As it turned out a new world record would be set that year by Wilson Kipsang of Kenya in a time of 2:03:23 so the Sub-2 marathon dream was beginning to look like a reality in my lifetime but for those of you that are more informed, taking another three minutes and some off that time is easier said than done and it would take someone very special to do it.

Meanwhile back on planet earth, were the earthlings working out their race strategies for a much more modest finish. I checked in to my hotel on the Friday before the race and began to suss out just how far away from the start the hotel was and to check out the finish area through the Brandenburg Gate and around the Reichstag.

The great thing about World Major marathons is that they take you right through the hearts of the city and around all the main historical buildings and the finishes are typically right next to great landmarks or in great parks. I decided to get registered on Friday so that I could spend Saturday taking in the sights and the atmosphere building around the course and the finish area.

The registration was a bit chaotic and took forever to get through. I was given a starting pen of D or F, or something, which seemed to be well back from the start but oddly there was a desk where you could go and appeal your starting pen and get one nearer to the start. They simply accepted my claim of a 2:45 attempt, and I was given pen A instead which would mean a starting pen closer to the Elites.

On the Saturday afternoon I booked a massage at the hotel for an hour to loosen up the legs and was lying on the massage table when a guy walked in and introduced himself and proceeded to oil up my legs and do whatever masseurs do. He seemed quite chatty, and it turned out he used to be the physio for Spartak Moscow, a big Russian soccer club.

We got chatting about his time doing that and he asked if I wanted a deep tissue massage or lighter and I said lighter as I was running the marathon tomorrow.

After ten minutes or so he said, "You're not a runner, are you?" This seemed a bit odd and a little harsh given I had almost one-hundred marathons under my belt, fifteen of which were Sub-3. "No, not really" I said "What makes you say that? "You were more of a soccer player I think when you were younger" he said. "Yeah", I said, "as a matter of fact that was all I did from a kid to about the age of thirty, how did you guess?" He said he could always tell what sport someone had grown up doing whether it was soccer, tennis, rugby, or athletics.

I guess most marathon runners, except for club runners, have come from some other sport where they need to run to keep fit to play their chosen sport and at some point, they cross over and running takes on a life of its own with its own goals and challenges and quests for trophies.

The start of the Berlin Marathon is very memorable as it is a long straight and wide start-grid running towards and around the towering Victory Column (Siegessaule) with Victoria, the Roman goddess of victory, staring down at you.

It is a very flat and open course where you can see what's ahead. It was quite a warm day but there were lots of shady street sections and I crossed halfway at 1:25:13 feeling 50/50 but surely enough in the bank to hold the second half barring a disaster.

I began to struggle with about five miles to go and I could feel the pace sliding and a couple of fast fun runners dressed as Mickey Mouse and Superman went past me which is normally a bad sign. I remember the last mile seeming to go on forever but suddenly the Brandenburg Gate came into view, with the finish 200 yards behind it.

The done deal feeling of another Sub-3 came into focus and I enjoyed the last few hundred meters knowing it was done. I finished in 2:58:00 and proceeded to the T-Shirts and medals queue with a satisfied smile on my face and the prospect of one of those German hot dogs.

I spent an hour or two basking in Sub-3 glory and taking in the sights at the finish before treating myself to an open top bicycle taxi back to the hotel for a well-earned bath before going straight to the airport and a flight to Barcelona for a business conference the following day.

With Sub-3 number sixteen in the bag and two more races planned for the year then the S3XX tattoo was being made ready.

24. Chicago Marathon 2013

Eggs and Air Jordans

Having nailed Berlin in 2:58 just a few weeks earlier, confidence of a Sub-3 Chicago was running high. I had read how the course was fast and flat so this should be a done deal. I had set up the usual fly-on Friday, register Saturday, run Sunday, flight home Sunday night. I had managed to get a hotel on the east side of the canal and within walking distance from the start and finish at Grant Park.

My sons were in their late teens and when they realised I was off to Chicago and the home of the Chicago Bulls, it dawned on them that I might be able to buy some Air Jordan shoes unavailable in the UK. I was given the task to find some Air Jordan Bred 4 shoes in their sizes and, being a great dad and a real man, this was clearly a challenge I had to deliver on.

After sorting out registration on Saturday morning I went to a general sports shop near to the hotel and they suggested I try some more 'independent' type shops as I was asking for something a bit more exclusive than what they typically stocked. They gave me the name of a 'cool independent shop' the other side of the canal, past Grant Park, and further south, so armed with the address and a city map I walked what felt like an eternity to find the shop.

I know what you're thinking, why didn't I simply phone shops from the hotel room and work it all out from there but when you have a whole day to kill and a family challenge to complete, then go in person. I would also need to get clearance from home that whatever I was about to buy was indeed the real thing or not. No room for knockoffs or the wrong shoe type here.

I don't know how far south down South Michigan Avenue I walked, and I don't remember the name of the boutique shoe store I finally found. It was a warm day and I had probably walked the best part of two miles but the store was stacked with shoes so this should be mission accomplished. Sadly, following a call home from the shop and the offering of something similar, it was clearly not the right shoe.

Happily, the store manager offered another place to try which was a similar boutique store but back north and what seemed to be nearer the hotel, so I yomped back the way I had come, back past Grant Park, past the hotel, west across the canal and north up Jefferson street, then left, right, left again up three blocks, across two more before I finally found the store I had been given.

It was probably a three mile walk back from the other store, but hey I have all day to kill on this task. Another dead end and another store suggested, which was back past the hotel again and south somewhere and after another couple of miles walking in the increasing heat of the day, I arrived at the third store and the third dead end for these shoes.

I had to give up on the Jordan 4 whatever quest and make my way to the hotel for a well-earned rest. I had been out walking for the best part of five hours, not great prep for a race the following day but if you can't handle five miles walking you certainly can't handle 26 miles running.

I lazed around the hotel for the rest of the day and set my alarm for a 5am wake-up call. The hotel was putting on an early breakfast and though I am not someone who can eat any breakfast on a race morning, going through the motions of it with all of the other runners is part of the pre-race ritual. The great thing about races in the USA is the sheer quantity and quality of food and drink they put on before and after an event. There is literally nothing they don't have if you want it.

I joined the throng of other runners working their way through all the buffet breakfast items available. I am fortunate to get just a coffee and a half a slice of toast down at this time of the morning but there was so much food I felt I should go a bit further.

I picked up a couple of eggs and put some bread on the rotating toaster thing they always have in a USA hotel breakfast setting. The eggs were in their shells and were cold so all I had to do was heat them up. I saw the queue for the microwave and with my coffee, toast, and eggs I joined the queue, smiling and nodding at the other runners and making polite conversation.

As my turn for the microwave approached, I realised I wasn't sure what was needed here. I put the two eggs on a plate and put them in the microwave and pressed a few timing buttons and hit Start. The queue behind me looked on. There was a pressured schedule to get breakfast done, back to bed for an hour and up and out to the start pens.

The eggs were still rotating, the light was still on, the whirring noise was still happening for what felt like an eternity. I put my coffee down to free up a hand when a muffled explosion seemed to be going on in the microwave.

The queue of athletes waiting to use it looked on anxiously. I tried to style it out thinking something traumatic may had befallen the eggs. The microwave pinged and fell silent so I opened the door and as if by magic the eggs had disappeared.

The inside of the microwave was completely covered with bits of white, shell, and egg yolk and I had written off the only microwave as unusable. I attempted to scrape some egg bits out to go on my toast and then knocked my coffee over and soaked the surrounding area of cereals and fruits and the floor beneath the microwave.

I hoped the runners in the queue weren't aiming for a fast time anyway and what's a cold breakfast now among friends. I went back to bed for an hour for a final sleep before up and go time. Breakfast had been the usual failure to get calories down, but eggs would never seem the same again.

Race day was perfect. A cool morning and an easy walk to Grant Park where the start area was located. The course was flat, and I had a red pen start (at the very front), so surely a Sub-3 finish and a relaxing flight home later that evening.

I made another schoolboy error at the start as I had decided to run with a new Ironman energy belt, and I stuck a couple of watered-down gels in it, so they were a bit chunky and heavy, and I didn't normally run with this sort of stuff hanging off me.

Within fifty yards of the start the belt was flapping up and down and it felt like I had two bags of sugar stuck to my backside. I kept adjusting the belt, but it just moved the flapping from one side of my waist to another so after a few hundred yards I jettisoned the extra baggage and threw it to the sidewalk.

Panic over, normal service resumed, settle down, settle in, get it done. I felt fine, the miles were rolling past but warning signs were already coming in with a 40:07 first 10k. This shouldn't be a problem but having analysed my results for this book in hindsight (see Chapter 28) then anything over 40 Minutes for a 10k would normally mean a failure.

At half-way I was still feeling OK, but something wasn't feeling right, and I crossed halfway in 01:27:49 which, again, based on analysis this is almost certainly too slow for my split personality.

By 30K the wheels were coming off and things started to go from maybe a near miss, to maybe still going under the London marathon qualify time for the next two years, to any sort of finish will do, to full walking mode and an embarrassing 3:28:38 finish. Not only did this look like the end of the Sub-3 dream it was also my worse finish for ten years since 2003.

Maybe the shine was starting to wear off, maybe I could blame it on the Air Jordan's and walking the length and breadth of Boston looking for them! Either way, the disappointment would be short lived as I was due to fly out of Chicago in just a few hours' time.

I grabbed an hour at the hotel bar waiting for a taxi to the airport and drowned my concerns with a beer or two. I reflected on what had just happened and how I had dropped back into the habits of a mid-race bonk. It wasn't as though I was unprepared as I had gone Sub-3 in Berlin just weeks before.

Having reviewed the Sub-3 results for all six World Majors in 2013 and ten years later in 2022/23 (See Chapter 26) then Chicago had less than 1,000 runners (2.3%) going Sub-3 in the year I ran it.

The good news was that redemption should come early with the New York marathon lined up in just three weeks' time and a final run of the year to complete the Big Six.

25. New York Marathon 2013

Just a Second!

The New York Marathon 2013 has a special place in the quest for a Sub-3 as it is the only marathon that has any pride of place in my home. I'm sure your assumption is that my home is covered in pictures of races, framed numbers, medals, and finisher shirts. You would be wrong.

There are several paintings and posters from Ironman races, but the only evidence of marathon running is a long fridge magnet I picked up at the New York Marathon whereby you can remove sections to depict your finish time. It was a Timex promotion. The magnet shows 3:00:01 and the reason it is there is because it represents the worst possible outcome of a Sub-3 attempt and is as near to the true definition between success and failure as you can get.

I have already covered a 3:00:33 finish Marathon in 2005. In that situation Sub-3 had been lost three miles from the finish. In this situation it was lost within 300 yards of the finish, and I am covering it so that it never happens to you. It appears on face value to be a one second miss, but it is of course a two second miss.

The New York Marathon is the biggest of the six majors at over 50,000 runners. It is also, in my opinion, the most restrictive as the only way to the start is via dedicated buses running from the city out to the Verrazano Bridge, which is fine except they want you at the start so early that you are leaving hotels at 5am and then hanging around the start area for hours in freezing weather.

You really must prepare for this and keeping warm right up to the start time is a key success factor. It is a flat course except the start is a long incline to the middle of the bridge and personally I hate races that have even the slightest of inclines right at the start. It's also exposed and can be quite windy so it's not the prettiest of starts but given the volume of runners I can fully understand why this works and that they also want the race to go through all five boroughs of New York.

I still vaguely remembered 1990 all those years ago and the memory of busing runners out to the start very early except this time I had gone to bed earlier and hadn't stayed out beyond midnight getting lashed up on Budweiser.

I had unexpectedly bonked at the Chicago Marathon a few weeks earlier so this was the last chance of the year to get things back on track. I had attempted to carry some gels (that weren't concentrated gels but were watered down) in Chicago but in a flimsy race belt that bounced around all over the place, so I had to throw them away just a few hundred meters into the race.

Armed with a new belt pouch, which wouldn't bounce around, would give me a chance of getting something down without gagging later in the race. They probably saved my race looking back. I had already Sub-3'd Tokyo, London, and Berlin that year. Boston is, in my opinion, not a flat marathon so it's not comparable and I had died in Chicago for whatever reason a few weeks earlier. New York was relatively flat but not as flat as Tokyo, London, Berlin, or Chicago as it had some inclines throughout the route that can feel like big hills when you are dying out there.

I took plenty of throw away clothes to the start to keep warm (this is the beginning of winter) and though it was annoyingly early, I managed to start within a meter or two of the start line, so the course clock was live and accurate and no real need to keep checking the wristwatch.

The playing of New York New York by Frank Sinatra was a nice touch before I engaged the headphones and shut off all outside noise save for the Sub-3 soundtrack.

As I've said, the start over the Verrazano bridge is an uphill start and very exposed to the elements so it's not an easy race to settle in to but coming down the other side you start to feel more super-human as the road starts to drop down. After two miles on the bridge, you are back on city terra firma with the start of the crowds for the run through Brooklyn and onto Queens.

If you're running to simply finish then you are probably taking in the sights and the crowd, if you're going Sub-3 you are shutting out the sights and the crowds and are simply focussed on making that halfway point in good time and good shape. I wasn't feeling great, but I wasn't feeling dead, so this was going to be one of those touch and go races. It could all fall apart in the second half.

141

I crossed half-way in 1:26:36 which was the right side of a Sub-3 split but the wrong side of previous races that year which had all gone Sub-3 and were all Sub-1:26 at the half. I didn't remember the course from 1990 and I hadn't done any research, so I wasn't ready for, or expecting, the Queensboro Bridge at mile fifteen which was another two mile drag with a long hard climb to the middle, very exposed with no crowd support despite them being shut out anyway by the Sub-3 soundtrack.

I do remember giving up on a Sub-3 at this point and starting to mentally settle for a 'good time', whatever that would be! The demons of Chicago were started to set in, and I began to question why I was still doing this anyway. I pressed on and the sight of Manhattan and the crowds the other side of the bridge seemed to deliver a bit of a calming effect.

The next few miles were though the Bronx and back into Manhattan and the clock suggested this was not over yet. I managed to get one gel down, then another, I felt sick, but I didn't gag it all back up. I attached myself to a couple of decent runners in front of me and I just ran right behind them. Like right behind them. Looking down at their shoes and hanging on in there. I didn't look up, or sideways or anywhere, just down at their shoes and I simply stayed with them for mile after mile after mile. I stopped checking my watch as it didn't matter.

The Sub-3 was probably gone but we were still well inside a Sub-3.05 so not the embarrassment of Chicago. I acknowledged the 23-mile, and 24-mile markers go by from under the brim of my cap, and I was feeling stronger. This had never happened before. Normally, the final miles were always simply holding on and dying, not speeding up. We approached 25 miles and now we are talking just the run up Central Park, right and right again and this pain is all over.

I knew it was a bit of a hill from Mile 25 to 26 before a right turn into the park for the last 400 meters or so as I had checked that out the day before. To my surprise I was still 9 or 10 minutes inside a Sub-3 at Mile-25, so this was more than just on. I felt good. I ran that hill up the left-hand side of the park in what felt like a good pace.

I wasn't checking times or watches. The task was simple. I made the top of the hill feeling good. I would have slowed down but this is easily on now, just hang on in there. I made the right turn into Central Park, and I knew we were talking just a few hundred yards to the finish line. This was a Sub-3, slam dunk, just enjoy the moment. I could now hear the race commentator and I knew the finish was just around the corner.

Then I thought I heard something along the lines of "Let's start the count down for three hours – 20, 19, 18, 17" over the sound system. Hang on a minute, surely, it's not that close.

I rounded the corner and could see the finish and the clock and could hear the countdown. I sprinted (in my mind) flat out to the line and I think I even did a chest out, head down, like they do in the 100 meters and the clock above was "2..." or was it "3...." I simply didn't know. Even if was "3...." my chip time would be better than my gun time, right? Well, I had started right on the start line so this benefit would be a second or two at most!

They don't give you a finish time at the finish, you don't get a print-out of your time and splits just your finisher goody bag, a medal, and some bananas (ugh!) and drinks and stuff. I picked that all up and made my way back through the crowds and to the hotel which took the best part of an hour and a half as they had cordoned off all the streets for security reasons following the Boston bomb back in April.

Was it Sub-3, was the only thing going through my mind and I tortured myself with 'no' I think the clock clicked "3" just when I went under it but then 'yes' surely I had at least three seconds chip-time vs gun-time and chip-time trumps gun-time. I got back to the hotel and decided to call my dad first as I knew he would have been tracking me on the race results site. This would be the moment of truth. Whatever came out of his mouth first would be success or failure.

"Hey Dad, only me, just checking in" I said, "Heya, well done, tracked you all the way, you must be really pleased with that?" he replied "Yeh, tough race but hung in there, wasn't sure the final time but." I paused waiting for the response "Three hours dead..........." he said but I don't remember what he said after "Three" as my heart sank as he didn't say "Two..........." If it had been 2:59:59 he would have said "Two............. blah" but all I heard was "Three...................". I could log-in to the results site but why would it be any different to what my dad had just said.

The official time was 3:00:01. You may be thinking this is a one second miss but clearly this is a two second miss and it might as well have been a ten-minute miss. That Fridge Magnet remains on our main home fridge to this day. London 2005 and a 3:00:33 finish seemed cruel, but this was as close as it gets.

As a footnote, I have taken four of the 2013 races (dropped the Chicago disaster and the Boston result) that were Sub-3 (except New York of course) and the distance split times. You can see the warning signs of New York early in the race.

RACE	TOKYO	LONDON	BERLIN	NEW YORK
YEAR	2013	2013	2013	2013
KM10	00:38:41	00:39:30	00:39:29	00:40:41
KM20	01:19:24	01:20:50	01:20:40	01:21:52
HALF	01:24:15	01:25:22	01:25:13	01:26:36
KM30	02:01:44	02:03:10	02:03:44	02:05:13
KM40	02:45:58	02:47:17	02:48:01	02:50:30
FINISH	02:56:24	02:57:17	02:58:00	03:00:01

The New York 10k split was 'OK' at 40 minutes plus but the other three were physically and psychologically better at Sub-40 pace. The 20k checkpoint was still OK at sub 1:22 but the other races were still holding a minute or more better at that checkpoint.

The half was 1:26:36 so again this should be fine for a Sub-3 with time in the bank at the half (I had been as late as 1.28 before). The 30k and 40k splits are both behind the other three Sub-3's that year. 40k is, more-or-less, 25 Miles in and I thought at this point I had plenty of time left to do this and I didn't overly push that last hill up to Central Park.

The reality is, I should have died on that hill rather than leaving too much to chance at the end. It's easy in hindsight and until I started writing this book I haven't looked back and analysed this stuff but it's becoming clearer now.

This should have been part of Sub-3 number 18 given one more achieved in 2014 but left me short of the S3XX target on just seventeen or S3XVII as a Sub-3 lifetime quest finish. Looking back at my 17 Sub-3's only two were achieved with half marathon splits later than 1:26 so New York was never really on the cards.

The others were between 1:20 and 1:25 so maybe the conclusion here is that if you are not comfortable with a neutral or negative split approach then you need to be training for a consistent and comfortable Sub 1:25 half marathon to pull this off. New York is a tougher race than the other three shown here (see previous table) so you will need even more in the bank at the halfway.

26. The Big Six - How they differ

On the face of it the 'Big Six' Abbot World Majors are similar. They are all big city marathons (Tokyo, Boston, London, Berlin, Chicago, New York), they are all big fields of thirty to fifty-thousand runners, they are all relatively flat, except for Boston and New York, but what sets them apart?

Well, the Boston marathon is 80% qualification and 20% charity, about 5% of London runners qualify, the rest being charity and ballot. There is a 10% chance of making the ballot in Berlin vs less than 4% in London.

Tokyo, Boston, and London are all within about 8 weeks of each other from late Feb to April with London being just six days after Boston. Berlin, Chicago, and New York are also all within about 8 weeks of each other from October to November.

The first Boston race was in 1897 so as the oldest one of the six, this has history bragging rights. Tokyo was first run in 2007 but was made a world major in 2013. London started in 1981, Berlin began in 1977 so the 2013 race was the 40th anniversary, Chicago began in 1977 and New York started seven years earlier in 1970.

New York (and now London) are the biggest with 50,000 runners and Boston the smallest with 30,000 runners. All marathons over-register the race based on a predicted percentage that will pull out through illness and injury. All courses are "flat" and fast though some are flatter and faster than others and some have sneaky little hills to catch you out (Boston, New York). I would say London, Berlin, Chicago, and Tokyo are the fastest in terms of being consistently flat and sheltered from wind and the sun due to most of the race being within high rise buildings and shady tree-lined streets.

But what about the chances of a Sub-3? Does that vary by course and has it changed much over time. So here are some comparisons between the six races I ran in 2013 and the same races ten years later (Chicago, Berlin and New York 2022 and Tokyo, Boston, London from 2023)

So first of all, the average finish time of all runners for Tokyo, London, Berlin, and Chicago is around 04:30 hours. They are the most similar in terms of their flatness and their mix of runners between qualification vs charity places. The average time for all runners in New York is 04:50 hours simply because the course is more hilly and less sheltered than the others.

The average time for all runners in the Boston Marathon is typically around 03:40 which is over an hour faster than New York and fifty minutes faster than the other four. But Boston is not a fast course compared to any of the others.

World records and PB's are typically not achieved in Boston due to the undulating hilly start, plus the notorious Heartbreak Hill at mile twenty where Eliud Kipchoge, the odds-on favourite for 2023 was brutally dropped from the front of the race to finish seven or eight minutes outside of his world record set in Berlin just six months earlier. The difference for Boston is simply the mix of runners that qualify versus those that get a place via charity or the ballot. The running field is simply quicker on average than the other majors.

Race	2013			2022/23		
	Finishers	Sub-3	Sub-3%	Finishers	Sub-3	Sub-3%
Tokyo	34,819	802	2.3%	36,536	1,954	5.3%
Boston	17,580	2,095	11.9%	26,600	4,188	15.7%
London	34,202	1,355	4.0%	48,634	3,034	6.2%
Berlin	36,568	1,482	4.1%	34,752	2,396	6.9%
Chicago	39,122	895	2.3%	39,420	2,072	5.3%
New York	50,062	775	1.5%	47,743	681	1.4%
Total	212,353	7,404	3.5%	233,685	14,325	6.1%

The table above compares then and now. Boston 2013 was the year of the bomb, where the race was stopped with just over 17,500 runners having crossed the finish line. Around 10,000 others were held back on the course and away from the finish area. It would include all runners that year going Sub-3 as the bomb went off an hour or more after that.

The size of the races haven't changed much over time except for London which now rivals New York with around 50,000 starters. The number and percentage of people going Sub-3 has increased markedly over the last ten years. Tokyo will have gained significantly after becoming a World major in 2013 with more 'serious' runners now opting to run it.

New York is clearly the toughest course to Sub-3 (Boston excepted) given only 1.5% seem to do it each year and well below 1,000 each year in total. Maybe my 03:00:01 time is feeling a bit better now. A massive

4,188 runners went Sub-3 in Boston in 2023 again due to the quality of the field and again why qualifying for Boston is an achievement in itself. Chicago is difficult for me to comment on as I completely blew up running it in 2013. On paper its fast but in 2013 at least only 2.3% went Sub-3 which is a surprising statistic for me. Maybe the search for those rare Air Jordan's all day and the eggs at breakfast fiasco weren't solely to blame.

So if it's a Sub-3 your are after then it has to be Tokyo, London, Berlin and maybe Chicago. If it's prestige you are after then Boston (but you will have to prove a good time to qualify) and if it's scenery, history and the arts or ease of running it then all six have their merits.

Berlin, Chicago, and Tokyo all start and finish in the city centre but importantly within easy reach of hotels near to the start and finish so logistically easier.

London, Boston, and New York start a long way outside the city, so you have the dilemma of staying near the start for an easier race morning schedule or near the finish for an easier beers and finish experience. Chicago is the earliest start time at 8.30am with Boston and London the latest at 10.00am. The later the start the more risk of warmer weather into the race.

Merch and medals vary depending on who is designing the finisher shirts each year. Races sponsored by Adidas have the best merch, by far, sorry, but they just do, and the Adidas Boston official race jackets are must-have merch items. Sponsors change from year to year and marathon to marathon, but Boston is always Adidas.

Goody bags are a thing of the past. You used to get a sack full of stuff at registration and another sack full at the finish, today it's a banana, a bottle of water, a bottle of non-alcoholic beer, and a load of promotional flyers.

They all have spectacular finishes through historic archways or in historic parks, except for Tokyo which is the most congested city on the planet.

For marathons in the USA, you can do it over three days if you are organised and prepared to fly home mid to late evening the same day as the race. Just make sure you don't have a complete meltdown or hit the wall harder than you were expecting.

There is talk of a seventh world major but because of Covid and cancellations they are now all over the place timewise. 2023 will be the first year in the last four years where they are all back to their 'normal' months of the year.

There may be a ban on certain types of shoes such as the Nike Alpha Fly's for the pro athletes. In my day the 'Super shoe' didn't exist though I did try something similar in 2015 (see Chapter 30). The percentage of people going Sub-3 has rising sharply since the introduction of these shoes in 2016 (see 2013 and 2023 comparison in the table previously).

Finally, if you manage to run all six World Majors then you get a massive medal the size of a dinner plate with all six medals welded together which you can use as a door stop.

27. Interview with Sub-2:30 finisher Immortality!

This book is about the challenge of Going Sub-3 and a semi-serious quest to do it and achieve legendary marathon status as an amateur, or hobby runner, or however you want to define that. Beyond that is achieving elite status and going under 2:45 which qualifies you for the elite start at any marathon and you will be rubbing shoulders with the marathon greats.

Elite begins at 2:45 and ends at 2:30, beyond that we are moving to immortality status.

Having invited a group of teacher colleagues to our house for dinner one evening, my wife mentioned that one of them "did some running" so I would at least have something in common with one of them in terms of conversation and I would be sitting next to him. I think that meant I wouldn't have anything intellectually in common with the rest of them and they could crack on and discuss all things teaching and she was hoping I wouldn't bore the poor running person to death with running and racing stories.

At least I could have the upper hand with the runner-type and could boast my Sub-3 credentials at some point into the conversation.

We got through the starter and halfway through the main course when the running conversation inevitably came up and it turned out he was a decent middle-distance runner and from what I could gather he seemed to be doing some serious county level championship type races at various tracks and meets around the country. He had run a few marathons but ultimately it wasn't his main thing.

He knew I was doing Ironman's and marathons from what my wife had told him, so he was interested in that and was impressed with how many races I had done, and he showed interest in the inevitable explanation of what an Ironman entails, and everything was going fine as desert was being served.

I asked what marathon's he had run, and it turned out to be a handful of London ones and of course I asked what his PB was and was waiting to hear a decent time like three-something when he said 2:29.

I nodded politely as my brain was trying to process what 2:29 meant. Perhaps he was a slow half marathon runner or something until it started to dawn on me that this was a full marathon time he was talking about. He mentioned it had been a few years ago and he had been getting slower since then, so he was focussing more on middle distance again.

I nodded beginning to wonder what getting slower meant. Having checked his times later, on the Power of 10 site, he meant a 2:32 followed by a 2:39 so yeah clearly this is getting slower, and I could understand his disappointment that he was no longer going Sub 2:30. And no, we are not talking half-marathons here.

Most of this book has been about the malarky of attempts at going Sub-3 and that time being the ultimate quest for most mortals running a marathon but given I now know someone who has gone Sub 2:30, that means inside the top 70 finishers of the London Marathon including the elite and professional men and women, then I thought it would be remiss of me not to talk to him and work out when he did it, how he did it, and why he did it.

He agreed and here's what he said in case you are feeling you may be closing in on that level. If I had gone Sub-2:30 it would be proudly tattooed on my neck but for him, it wasn't necessarily the greatest sporting achievement of his life so for the purposes of interview I will refer to him as Modest Martin (MM).

ME: So, what's your background in terms of sports and running before the Sub-2:30?

MM: Mostly 3k, 5k, 10k, half-marathons and cross-country type championships through to my late twenties, early thirties.

ME: What sort of times are we talking?

MM: Sub-32 10k's, fifteen-minute 5k's and Sub-1:10 half marathons.

ME: What made you decide to run a marathon?

MM: I've only run a handful of marathons, all London, and you can qualify for the London Marathon based on a half-marathon championship time and I had run a couple of halves at 1:09.

(That was news to me, so I looked it up and, in case you're wondering, the Championship Qualify for London for Men is ether a proven Sub-2:40 Marathon or a proven Sub-1:12:30 half marathon! At least they give you the extra thirty seconds here!)

ME: So, when did you run your first full and what was the time?

MM: 2001 or 2002 and 2:39.

ME: So, you're second marathon is 2004 and this is the 2:29 year. What was the run up to it? What time where you targeting? What was different and what were the tactics? Basically what was the deal here?

MM: Looking back I was in the shape of my life because I had gone the longest, fastest, fittest period of races without injury and I was weighing in at my lowest weight ever.

ME: So, weight was important?

MM: Very, not an unhealthy weight-loss programme or anything like that just the sheer volume of running and races without injury, whatever you are eating your weight must come down.

(I thought about Mystic Chris and his weight loss tactics to go Sub-4!)

ME: So, from what to what?

MM: I weighed in around 58kg for that marathon, down from a typical weight of 60-61kg – but I'm only 5' 6".

ME: And were you specifically targeting Sub-2:30 or just let's see how it goes?

MM: No, specifically Sub-2:30 was the plan, nothing over that would be a success. I figured I was probably capable of a 2:27 or 2:28 but that would be a risk.

ME: A risk, how?

MM: Well like you trying to go Sub-3, you will know that you are probably capable of 2:50 but if you go out at that pace you risk a 3:01 finish vs a 2:59 finish" (that sounded familiar!)

ME: So, what was the mile pace plan?

MM: 5:42

(Thinking now about my PB with Elmbridge Guy and his 6:10 plan and how slow that now feels).

ME: That was precise. Surely you can't calculate that math in your head mile by mile.

MM: No but when you are running dozens of 5k's and 10k's every year you instinctively know what that pace is and there are 5k and 10k markers on the course, so they are as, if not more, important than the mile-by-mile check-in.

ME: So, would that be a negative, neutral, or positive split personality and pace?

MM: Positive. So, running the first half quicker to offset a possible second half slowdown. I went through halfway at 1:14:30.

ME: So just thirty seconds in the bank saved up to offset any second half slowdown.

MM: Yes, at this pace you can't be building more than that or you are back in the risk and fail factor.

ME: At what point do you let go of the watch and the clock?

MM: About 20 miles is when you start to lose interest in the clock, or your brain can't process what's going on anymore"

(Roger that, at least something is the same for a Sub-3)

ME: How do you know you won't lose that thirty second advantage?

MM: The runners around you.

ME: Dropping off?

MM: Yes, you're not running any faster, it's just others are dropping off the pace.

ME: So, they are saying goodbye to a Sub-2.30?

MM: I guess, there aren't many runners out there for company from the start, so you get familiar with them early on and it's a quiet acknowledgment as one-by-one they drop off and you hope it's not coming for you.

ME: What about nutrition, drinks, gels, Cornish pasties?

MM: None with you, just drinks on the course, no point being lighter and then carrying gels for extra weight.

ME: Running technology? Watches, heart rate monitors, magnetic bracelets?

MM: None, there were no Garmin's and stuff back then, just a watch and the official race clock and on the Championship Start I was given Band 1, but you are still behind the professional runners and a few others, so it was about nine seconds between the watch and the clock. You just know instinctively what your race pace is as you've done it time and time again at 5k and 10K race level.

ME: Did you wear any fancy shoes? (Thinking off my 2015 London marathon and my fancy shoe blow-up).

MM: Not really, Asics generally.

ME: Anything else you can remember and share to anyone reading this who might be considering a Sub-2.30?

MM: The taper before the race. I had a school ski-trip two weeks before the race, so I didn't do any running that week and the week before the race was some light jogs. I wouldn't normally have that amount of time not doing fast training runs and I thought that could be a problem. It wasn't so I think it doesn't matter what you do with two weeks to go as whatever you have done up until then is your down payment for the race, some people still go out running the night before the race but it's not buying anything more by then.

According to The Power of 10 website, MM was ranked 46th of ALL GB athletes for his 2004 time of 2:29:30 for all marathons run that year. His split times were 1:14:30 for the first half and 1:15:00 for the second. That's as near to a neutral split as you can get, and the discipline needed to do that is mind boggling.

For the handful of immortals out there who have gone Sub-2:30 then hats off and God speed. I guess this book is of little interest to you but for the rest of us it's nice to know there is always another level to get to.

28. Doing the Splits

Your Split Personality

I mentioned the importance of split times based on four races in 2013 that were all Sub-3 or within one second of that. I was never a runner obsessed with this, but the initial mile splits clearly count and the 5k and 10k checkpoints are critical if you are on a fast time schedule.

The key is to work out what your split personality is and break down your checkpoints from there. You need to know off by heart, your mile or kilometre pace, your 5k and 10k expectations and most importantly of all, your halfway target.

The halfway target determines your split personality and whether you should pace the first half faster than the second, slower than the second, or the same as. A serious Sub-3 like the PB I ran in 2008 in 2:46:30 required a friendly pacemaker (Elmbridge Guy) who I met at the start line and was adamant about 6:10 mile splits to go Sub-2.45.

We (or he) hit them on the nose throughout the race right up until half way, for me at least, when I slipped off the pace by a few seconds and paid the price of not going 2:45 as a result. He had even been specific about having to be at Mile 24 by 2:30 or a Sub-2:45 is off and I got there about 2:31.

So specific splits do matter if you are aiming for Immortality and the Elite qualifying time and that is a different league altogether where there is much less room for error.

There are three split personality types.

(1) Negative – pace the second half faster than the first half so don't build a time bank to offset a slowdown or a meltdown later but include the need to increase your pace from halfway.

(2) Positive – pace second half slower than the first half so build a time bank before halfway to offset a slowdown or a meltdown in the second half or,

(3) Neutral – pace a perfect 1:30 first half and a perfect 1:30 second half.

For me it must be a high positive. For a Sub-3, I only felt compelled to check the watch, or the clock, every mile or two for the first eight or nine miles, and make sure I crossed the half-way line four or five minutes inside 1:30.

Given a marathon is essentially four back-to-back 10k's and imperial marathons (UK and USA) tend to have kilometre markers every 5k then this is also a key checkpoint and requires less maths the further into the race you get. Maybe a check here and there after halfway but close the pain off, stay with the pace and check again with two or three to go and hope the Sub-3 pacemakers don't sidle past in the meantime.

I only used to keep a record of my Sub-3 marathons after a while, but I have managed to find full time splits for some of my road marathons since 2003 onwards and so, as research for the book, I tried to analyse them based on the table of results shown.

Not all marathons provide full splits but here are a few pointers if you are a negative split personality. If you can't comfortably go Sub-40 for the first 10k split, then the chances are you will fail the task. I did manage to do it twice being over 40 minutes but for the two near miss Sub-3's I was guilty of going over 40 minutes for the first 10k. Going Sub-40 for the first 10k is not a guarantee of a Sub-3 but going over is typically a no-no.

Holding sub 1:26 at halfway was almost, but not always a Sub-3 finish guarantee. Going over 1:26 was almost, but not always a guarantee of not making it. London 2015 was an anomaly as that was the year my legs blew up just before Tower Bridge for wearing silly shoes.

London 2011 looks like a blow up given a Sub-40 first 10k and sub 1:25 half and a 3:01:54 finish. I don't remember what happened there but clearly a screw up. Having checked the race weather for 2011 it was "unusually hot" at 20C, and heat is my main nemesis. Even Cracknell went 3:03:56. Hills and heat and that's game over for me at least.

So, conclusion is, if you are a positive split personality and you want some pre-race training and practice then you need to be a comfortable Sub-40 10k runner. If you do a few halves beforehand aiming for Sub-1:26 finishes you could pull off a Sub-3 full marathon. I'm not a coach or an expert but I have run a lot of these things in all weathers and cities, so I hope this gives you some food for thought.

COURSE	YEAR	KM10	KM20	HALF	KM30	KM40	FINISH
LONDON	2003	00:42:31	01:28:09	01:33:27	02:19:09	03:20:22	03:32:53
LONDON	2004	00:44:57	01:31:09	01:36:12	02:17:48	03:05:57	03:15:50
LONDON	2005	00:40:22	01:22:35	01:27:07	02:05:53	02:50:51	03:00:33
DUBLIN	2005	00:41:22		01:28:09			02:58:48
OC LA	2006	00:39:06		01:30:41			03:08:12
LONDON	2006	00:39:10	01:19:29	01:23:55	02:00:36	02:43:29	02:53:00
OC LA	2007						02:53:21
LONDON	2007	00:38:29	01:18:06	01:22:27	01:58:20	02:41:38	02:51:14
OC LA	2008						02:50:03
LONDON	2008	00:38:13	01:16:58	01:21:06	01:55:57	02:37:13	02:46:30
LONDON	2009	00:37:30	01:16:29	01:20:49	01:56:26	02:37:55	02:46:59
DUBLIN	2009	00:39:24		01:24:34	02:01:34		02:55:28
LONDON	2010	00:38:50	01:20:28	01:25:05	02:04:05	02:50:02	02:59:52
DUBLIN	2010	00:39:11		01:23:31	02:00:00		02:52:57
TOKYO	2011	00:38:33	01:19:09	01:23:52	02:02:36	02:48:03	02:58:20
LONDON	2011	00:39:07	01:20:13	01:24:54	02:04:03	02:51:09	03:01:54
DUBLIN	2011			01:25:22			02:57:39
DUBLIN	2012	00:40:57		01:27:27			02:58:58
TOKYO	2013	00:38:41	01:19:24	01:24:15	02:01:44	02:45:58	02:56:24
BOSTON	2013	00:40:21	01:22:03	01:26:43	02:10:25	03:06:57	03:18:45
LONDON	2013	00:39:30	01:20:50	01:25:22	02:03:10	02:47:17	02:57:17
BERLIN	2013	00:39:29	01:20:40	01:25:13	02:03:44	02:48:01	02:58:00
CHCAGO	2013	00:40:07	01:22:47	01:27:49	02:11:29	03:15:19	03:28:38
NEW YORK	2013	00:40:41	01:21:52	01:26:36	02:05:13	02:50:30	03:00:01
LONDON	2014	00:39:03	01:20:18	01:24:51	02:03:02	02:47:36	02:57:36
LONDON	2015	00:39:50	01:23:39	01:28:55	02:12:32	03:04:03	03:14:14

Putting this into practise recently I spoke to a woman in the 18-34 category who was running London 2023 as her first ever marathon in just a few days' time. She was aiming for a Sub-3:30 finish to get a Boston Qualify time so full marks for ambition vs "I just want to finish". She had completed some 20-mile training runs and to my surprise she was feeling comfortable with running a negative split as she felt she was running faster after halfway during training runs though she hadn't really measured how much faster, and she hadn't gone the full distance as yet. Given men are 10-15% stronger and faster on average than women then a Sub-3:30 attempt here is bordering on a Sub-3 for men so even more respect.

We discussed race tactics, and her plan was to go out at 8-minute mile pace for the first half which after a quick calculation is 1:44:48 at the half which would certainly need a neutral split at best or a negative split at worst to do it. That's just twelve seconds in the bank.

I suggested she might want to go out a bit quicker at say 7:50 mile pace and I tracked her progress during the race. She crossed halfway in 1:44:48. No kidding. Like within a second of her planned race pace. She finished in 3:37:14 as the fatigue in the second half of the race began to eat into her pace (as it does for most runners) but even so a pretty amazing first attempt and maybe a need to think about a positive split strategy next time.

Afterwards she explained that her GPS watch had her down as a 3:35 finish and 1:43:10 at the half so nearly two minutes faster than her chip time. The race clock on the course can't help here unless you are literally starting on the start line so maybe ditch the GPS and get a standard old Timex or Casio.

By happy coincidence, the ultimate negative and positive split times ever recorded in marathon running history have happened within six months of each other. The first at the Berlin Marathon 2022 by Eliud Kipchoge in a new world record and the second by Kelvin Kiptum six months later in the London Marathon where a new course record was set along with the second fastest time in marathon history.

There are two particularly interesting things about this.

Firstly, both men ran a Sub 1-hour first or second half of the race for the first time ever, meaning the Sub 2-hour marathon barrier could be broken in my lifetime but secondly, whereas Kipchoge ran a positive split, Kiptum ran a negative one.

This is insanely fast and hopefully someone one day will be compelled to write a new memoir 'Sub-2 A quest for the impossible'.

I'll leave you to decide which of these two race splits you find the most impressive. Berlin is a faster course than London so the finish times are pretty much equal.

Runner	Race	Year	1st half	2nd half	Finish
Kipchoge	Berlin	2022	00:59:01	01:02:08	02:01:09
Kiptum	London	2023	01:01:40	00:59:45	02:01:25

Kipchoge has run a Sub 2-hour marathon but under artificial conditions with teams of pacers, laser beams from a car tracking the exact pace, special shoes, and a perfect flat loop course somewhere in Vienna. The times above are under 'normal' race conditions.

29. I don't know where you find the time!

I did say this book is not a How to Guide. It's simply how I did it. If I had a pound for the number of times someone has said "I don't know where you find the time?" then I would be rich. I developed a solid retort by saying that all I needed was fifteen minutes of their time to work out where they did have the time to do this, regardless of how big their career was or how much family time they needed to spend. They were simply making different time choices.

Question 1 would always be "Do you play golf?" If the answer was yes then game over as a typical round of 18-hole golf takes at least five hours, plus all the time toing and froing from the driving range so it's a choice, golf or Ironman and you chose golf.

Question 2 would be around hobbies "Do you do much reading?" If yes, then how much. So you choose to read whereas I choose to run.

Question 3 "Do you get the train to work?" If yes, then why not cycle and so on.

For me, it was not about *balancing* career, sport and family time as separate things but *blending* and merging them into one big thing with no time spent or wasted on anything else.

A two-week holiday with the family in the sun would typically include ten or more half marathons (one each day before going out to dinner), two or three long bike rides of over one-hundred miles (bikes would travel with us or be kept at the destination permanently) and five or six two-to-three-kilometre sea swims up and down the coast (just before lunch).

My wife would be happy laying in the sun reading, my kids were pre-teens and would happily play in the sand and I would still have plenty of time to swim with them, build castles and play beach ball games throughout the day.

This is clearly intensive stuff but if you build your sport around your life and you religiously do something every day regardless of what your work or personal life schedule is you may surprise yourself as to how much you can pack in.

Throughout that ten-year period or so, I was cycling twenty or more miles to work and back four or five days a week along the river tow path and putting in the odd 5k or 10k swim race here and there, plus half Ironman's and various ultra runs like London to Brighton cross country and Town to Tring, not to mention cycling to Northampton and back to visit parents.

Business trips to Tokyo for three or four days would include a 12-mile run every morning, trips to conferences in Europe and the USA would always have a 12-13 mile run every morning. Working out of a Neuss head office in Germany would include a 12-13 mile run along the Rhine every morning. While colleagues had breakfast, I went running. Breakfast was a five-minute pick up of bacon slices and coffee and straight to work. Every day involved a run or cycle or lake swim of some sort with weekends reserved for whatever race had been scheduled.

For one year of my working life, I was based in an office next to Waterloo station. I lived about twelve miles away on the river near Hammersmith Bridge, so I chose to run to work along the river and get the tube home or get the tube to work and run home. The office had a shower so no problem and sometimes I would run in and run back.

Some people would often say they would use the time on the train to read. Fine, I would say I don't know where you get the time to read as I simply don't have enough time in the day to run and read. I would ask where their parents lived and how often they visited them. I would suggest maybe they cycle next time and ask their wife or husband to drive the kids in the car and meet them there, you can choose to drive for two hours or cycle for seven or eight.

If you have an understanding partner you can do this. I still had plenty of time to take the kids to rugby and football training at weekends and I never missed a parent's evening, or a school play, or a birthday party.

I was never away for long and would keep race time to as short a time as possible. For Endurance life races I would drive four or five hours from work on a Friday evening and pull into a hotel or B&B late that night. The race start was typically 7am and after a four-to-five-hour marathon or ultra-run I would drive straight back to London and be home early evening. For one of my son's school plays I took my seat next to my wife five minutes before the lights went down, and the play started.

Family trips to Cornwall would also have bikes thrown in to break the week up into running and biking. The two-kilometre evening walk to the Pandora Pub for dinner along the estuary would mean a swim for me and a walk for the family. We would arrive at the same time, and I would change in the pub toilets from wetsuit to shorts and T-shirt.

Even a gym membership is questionable. If it takes you 15 minutes to drive to the gym, 15 minutes to get ready, one hour on the treadmill, and 30 minutes to change and get back home then you have lost an hour not gained one. You could have gone out for a two-hour run instead.

So, whoever you are, whatever you do, wherever you live, you do have the time to train for a Sub-3 marathon as you all have at least ten to twenty hours a week that you choose to spend time on other things like reading, golfing, driving, relaxing, sitting on a beach when you could be swimming the length of it. This is probably the subject of another book, but I challenge you to challenge yourself.

In 2005, I got talking to a guy who was racking his bike next to me for the Vitruvian Half Ironman near Rutland Water. As it turned out he explained he worked for a Leadership and Development consultancy built around sport which I found interesting as I was always looking for new ways to develop my management team and the sales teams in particular.

He gave me his details and a week later I met the company founder and we agreed to put the company leadership team and the sales team through a performance management course with a sport psychology theme to it.

They brought along Olympic gold medallists as key-note speakers as well as professional football and basketball players to explain the link between sport performance and business performance.

They worked on nutrition, attitude, engagement, self-motivation, team dynamics and a variety of other things. We even ended up on a three-day training session in the Lake District (I managed to get a 12-13 mile run in before dinner up and down the infamous Hard Knott pass).

Before we joined the course, we had to complete a basic life-style questionnaire and identify what our goals and expectations of the course and programme should be. I managed to find my questionnaire response from back then (Feb 2006) and this had included a specific goal around career, sport, and family time based on a daily training diary I had been keeping for a year prior to that.

Looking back, maybe this does seem a little bit obsessive, but it kept me focussed for years after,

Age: 45

Job Title: General Manager (UK, Eire, & Nordics)

Interests: Family, Work, Triathlon

A memorable moment: Leaving the USA

Things I love: Family, Work, Triathlon

Things I can't stand: Political hypocrisy, Govt waste, weak Journalism.

When it comes to sport: I love it/live for it

Things that are important to me: Family, Work, Triathlon

Food I enjoy: Beans on Toast, Marmite Slices, Tuna Fish, Chips, Cereals, white meats, pasta, pies, minced beef.

Food I don't eat: Fish (except Tuna), fatty meats, red meats,

My preferred learning style: All below

- Listening
- Discussing
- Group exercises
- Q & A

My expectations for the program:

That it enables me to achieve four high-level objectives (two business, two personal) at the same time, all of which require high levels of time and energy input.

Estimated time/week required – Work (50 hours), Ironman (12 hours), Family Time (46 hours), Sleep (60 hours)

1) Maintain 'Business-As-Usual'– includes new Nordic BU!
2) Implement fundamental cultural change within UK business.
3) Achieve Sub 11 Ironman, Sub 3:30 IM Marathon, Sub 2:50 Marathon
4) Maintain 'Quality Family Time' and not cannibalize with above.

In case and you may be wondering how those goals worked out, well in terms of a career, I lasted another eight years with that company and I ended up running the European business, so the work hours needed to do that increased over time as did the amount of travel to places all around the world. I am still happily married, and the kids are still talking to me. I kept the daily training diary going for four years and in case you are interested in how that went then I found it on an old laptop.

AVE/MINS	2005		2006		2007		2008	
PER WEEK	TOTAL	CALS	TOTAL	CALS	TOTAL	CALS	TOTAL	CALS
SWIM	43	518	25	301	57	678	22	263
BIKE	380	3,803	532	5,317	449	4,488	440	4,402
RUN	168	3,367	302	6,048	334	6,677	428	8,560
TOT	592	7,687	859	11,666	839	11,843	890	13,225

So, from the Performance Management Company course the training target for 2006 was 11 hours (660 Minutes) a week across the triathlon disciplines but this got smashed with up to 860 minutes a week on average as the obsession (dedication) to Ironman increased and the amount of running started to go up significantly based on the high schedule of marathon races now that the Sub-3 barrier had been broken and the target of Sub 2:50 had also gone with it.

By 2008 this had risen to almost 15 hours per week and an average weekly calorie burn of around 13,000 calories based on my basic formula of calorie burn by activity type. For 2008, the shortest training week was 440 minutes (7.3 hours) and the longest at 1,500 minutes (25 hours) which was a week that included almost 1,200 minutes of cycling.

This is a book about running and not triathlon and I did initially say that my running times were improving based on running less. That was probably the case initially as swimming and cycling time was absorbed but on reflection the amount of running was increasing more over time than swimming and cycling. I separated the running numbers out and converted them to hours and compared 2005 through 2008 and it's pretty clear how much the running hours per year increased over time from 150 hours in 2005 to over 370 hours in 2008 which works out at over seven hours average per week. The balance of swimming and cycling enabled more running intensity without injury. The lowest running week in 2008 was 3.3 hours and the highest was 13.2 hours. Only one week in 2008 was a rest week with zero running hours and only five weeks in four years (2005-8) were rest weeks with no running. The impact on marathon PB (see Chapter 36) was 2005 (02:58:48), 2006 (02:53:00), 2007 (02:51:14), and 2008 (02:46:30)

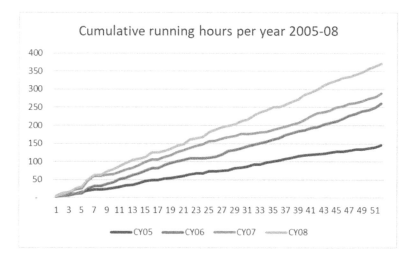

Cumulative running hours per year 2005-08

I have said before that you need to build your sport around your life not your life around your sport but what does that mean? Well I tried to explain it earlier that it is not being about *balancing* work, life and sport but *blending* them into one big thing with no time wasted on anything else even down to the Gym membership[example earlier.

I recently stumbled across something on Linked-In by Daniel Abrahams that talks about different types of work-life balance and maybe he is better at explaining this than I am. He provides some pictorial examples (see below) and explains it as follows:-

"Balance isn't about equal parts. It's about finding where you feel balanced. For some, balance may involve working long hours for a few weeks or months and then taking a longer break to recharge. Others may prefer to work shorter days and take frequent breaks throughout the day to pursue personal interests or hobbies. And for some, balance may mean taking a step back from work altogether to focus on their health or family. The key is to find what fits your own individual needs and priorities. Balance is where YOU feel balanced."

For most of us work comes first as that is normally how the bills get paid. Typically as you rise through the management ranks there are more and more things that seek to take up your limited time and work is no longer a 9-5 issue no matter how much you hope it would be.

When a family arrives on the scene, more time needs to be devoted to that. If sport is a key part of your life and you want to get better at it then more time needs to be devoted to that. And you need to sleep. Something has to give unless you find ways to blend or balance these things together and I have given some examples of how to that. There are dozens more I could have used but to maintain a high level of sporting achievement whilst holding down a high-level job and a growing family requires an understanding partner and a different way of doing things.

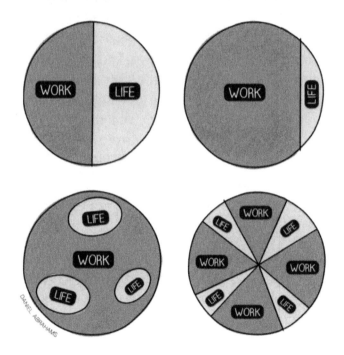

Despite the level of training I was doing, I was pretty much injury free and at my lightest. Time spent training (on the road, on the bike, in a boat or in the water) is clearly and obviously key to going Sub-3 but the biggest benefit is the impact it has on the weight to power ratio.

Although weight is clearly a factor in the equation somewhere, I never used to weigh myself nor care too much as I pretty much always burned enough calories to compensate for what I ate and drank.

I did start to become more interested in this as time went on and I was surprised to find the ideal weight for a 5 feet 10 inches male was between 149-183lbs and typically weighing in around 12 stone (173lbs) put me well into the higher end of that scale. I started thinking about how to get my weight down. I set a target of 160lbs and started to measure it on a daily basis.

I bought a diary, every year, with one of those year planners over two pages and wrote my weight down every morning to monitor it. The first weigh in was 173lbs on January 1st. I was surprised how much your weight can fluctuate by as much as five or six pounds during a day.

If you weighed in at night or in the morning or at mid-day you could get three very different readings, so the only valid reading had to be first thing in the morning after a dump, before a cup of coffee and that was the official weigh in.

The simple fact of writing it down religiously every day was enough to keep it under control. If you had a day where you had not done much exercise, then don't have a big evening meal. Try and eat before 7pm and you would be rewarded the following morning with a better weigh in.

I wasn't overweight to start with, so this is not exactly a candidate for a front cover Men's Health story but just to have a mental fix on it was enough for it to start to fall slowly but surely over the months that followed.

I eventually started weighing in at 159-160 lbs and I was noticeably gaunter as people who hadn't seen me for a while would comment on how ill I looked. I think they meant healthy but ill was a good enough measure for me.

I used to use lbs vs kg because I felt you could see changes more quickly and more precisely although 160lbs is not exactly a great weigh in for a marathon runner, as that's still a stone or two more than an ideal running weight for someone of my height, but to get below this would have required some sort of draconian diet plan and that for me was not a price worth paying.

I kept a daily record on a spreadsheet for a few years and averaged my weekly weigh-ins. There were a handful of weeks where I didn't weigh in such as holiday.

There's no point in doing all this if you must give up drink and fish and chips and all the luxuries of life. No point at all. Still, for me it simply came down to a diary, a pen and set of scales and being conscious of it on a daily or regular basis.

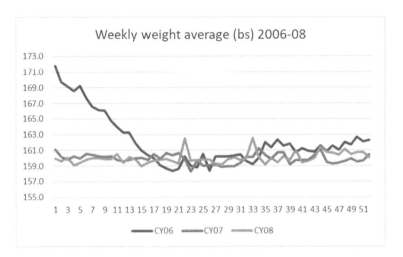

Weekly weight average (bs) 2006-08

CY06 — CY07 — CY08

Clearly my weight didn't come down simply because I recorded it every morning. It came down because of the switch to Ironman in 2003 and the increase in activity hours per week by cycling to work every day, long runs, and races most weekends and the odd crazy distance lake-swim (5k's and 10k's).

Running hours increased significantly from 2006 onwards as explained earlier but the daily focus on weight added to the incentive of spending more time on activity and not missing sessions due to apathy or something better on the TV. Weight and Time were working together as the key to maintaining long term Sub-3 ready fitness. Sub-160 (lbs) was a daily concern.

I was never, or rarely, injured throughout that whole ten-year period (2003-13) doing that level of training. I don't remember missing a race or putting in a bad time due to injury. Having interviewed Modest Martin about his Sub 2:30 marathon time in 2004, he said a similar thing in that he was in the shape of his life and at his lowest ever weight due to a long period of un-injured training.

Mystic Chris had attempted some rather eccentric short term weight loss tactics with some dodgy obesity pills and a colonic irrigation session, neither of which worked, but he did put his PB down to being at his lowest weight ever due to a period of sustained uninjured training.

Whether you are me at 5' 10" weighing in at 72kg, down from 80kg, or Modest Martin at 5' 6" weighing in at 58kg, down from 61kg or Mystic Chris at 5' 7" weighing in at 59kg, down from 75kg, we all had one thing in common. Our fastest ever times were at our lowest ever weights. Clearly there is a world of difference between Martin and Chris PB's (2:39 vs 3:47) with similar heights and weights but there is a common theme here.

So, although this is not a self-help 'How To" book, and I am no expert, the key to Sub-3 probably does come down to your weight on race day driven by sustained injury free training. The only question is how to get there without resorting to diet pills.

For me it was about intense but varied training with swimming and cycling to enable increased running. For Martin it was about increased running but staying injury free – the risk of injury goes up the more running you do but in my case the risk of injury came down as I was offsetting increased running with other stuff. Running is the most efficient way of losing weight as it burns the most calories, but it comes with a higher risk of injury.

30. London Marathon 2015

If the shoe fits don't wear it

The start of every major marathon involves a quick check on who is wearing what shoes and who bought them new from the Expo the day before. I realised back in the early days that Asics and Saucony seemed to be the shoe of choice among a large proportion of those starting in the Sub-3 start pen, so I went with Asics and went on to realise that there is more than one shoe type and lots of decisions around flat or supported.

I even had someone do one of those videos of you on a treadmill while you are running which made me feel sick and woozy when they played it back as you realise how much stress legs are put under when running at pace, so I was pretty sold and bought Gel Kayano's year in year out for fifteen years or more at around £120-£130 a pop. I bought a new pair the day before the Orange County Marathon in 2008 at the Expo. I walked them in the day before and ran a 2.50 the day after so the myth around not running in brand new shoes is not a solid one.

For London 2015 I was beginning to think of another Sub-3 on the journey towards the S3XX Tattoo having done seventeen and the last one being the year before in London. The shoes were up for replacement, so I wandered onto the various websites to order the Gel Kayano's as usual. I thought I would have a browse around to confirm the choice when I noticed something new, well new to me, as I didn't normally stray from making a quick purchase. The Gel-Hyper Speed-6. For serious runners only. Well, that must be me then! The racing flat of choice (Gel Kayano's aren't flat), suitable for halves and 10k's and marathons for Elite runners at 2:30 pace and below 60kg in weight.

OK, a few alarm bells there given I am packing 75-80kg nowadays and Elite is a bit of a stretch, and we are not talking middle distance. But hey, I'm the guy who has run brand new shoes in the past and maybe I needed something extra this year for that eighteenth Sub-3. The S3XX Tattoo was suddenly becoming clearer and bigger and maybe one on each calf.

Not too pricey, about the same as normal. Let's get a pair. Hell no, let's get two pairs! A few hundred quid on PayPal later and these puppies are being shipped already, clearly lots of stock!

So, two or three days later am I greeted by a package in the hallway but clearly something is wrong as the package is so light, they must have shipped one pair instead of two. Never mind, one will do for now, so I eagerly ripped the package open only to discover that there were indeed two pairs of these suckers. My god these are light I thought. I quickly tried them on, they fit like a glove, surely a Sub-3 guaranteed and who knows if I feel good, this could be another attempt at Sub-2:45.

I ran a few short loops in them over the coming weeks alternating between them and the old Kyano's until the big day approached. I made sure people had a good view of them on the underground to Embankment station and the train out to Blackheath. From there the walk to the Good for Age start and throughout the pre-race rituals in the holding area I noted I was clearly the only one wearing these Cinderella's.

Too late losers, these are the new breed, the Vapor Fly's before their time, the difference between Paula and Crawler. Now here they are on my feet, standing right on the Red start line as destiny beckoned. Sub-3 number 18 should be done and dusted and in the bag.

The first 5k was like clockwork and on time, maybe under time, could they even deliver a negative split. Through 10k, well under forty minutes, looking good, feeling strong. Cutting past the Cutty Sark, I glanced admirably down at the pounding Hyper-Speed 6's and maybe they weren't running shoes after all, maybe I was running in bare feet like Zola Budd. The ultimate weightless shoe and I'm the only wearing them.

I scorned and 'smugged' at those running around me in their concrete laden Kyano's and Saucony's and I began putting them to the sword, one by one, as I cut majestically through the field. Through fifteen kilometres and on towards the twelve-mile marker and the big feeding station before the right turn onto Tower Bridge and the run down to the halfway marker and still well inside a 1:25 halfway split time.

A slight slowing of pace at the 12-Mile feed station to take on water and............. boom! A complete seizure of both legs. No warning, no gradual feeling of a looming issue, just boom. Like a car with no gas, a bike with no chain, a fish without water, just seizure throughout the back of both hamstrings. Race over, red card, DNF, grounded.

This was serious. I had been injury free for my entire sporting life save for a broken arm, collar bone and the odd concussion playing rugby, but this felt very different. I staggered around a while and tried to walk it off but nothing. I felt my legs thinking a vein had come out or something but just numbness. A complete shutdown.

I stopped and drank some more water as the Kyano's and Saucony's filed pass me at pace carrying those still inside a Sub-3. Maybe I can walk it off but it's looking more like heading for the tube station on the other side of Tower Bridge and calling it a day.

I managed to walk across the Bridge, and I managed to convince myself not to settle for a DNF and to make the turn right towards Canary Wharf which would mean I would have to finish the race.

I started thinking of a finish, any type of finish would be a victory now though any thought of a Sub-3 was complete curtains. I felt better after walking a mile or two but not so much better as to push for anything, so I resorted to a jog 500 yards, walk 500 yards approach and to my credit I crossed the line in 3:14 which was good enough to qualify for a Good for Age slot again.

I could have DNF'd but didn't and I regard this as an honorary Sub-3 if that might count which of course it doesn't. My legs felt better by the end, and I ambled off on the tube having lived to fight another day.

About two days later in the evening after a shower and walking around in my underpants my wife exclaimed "Have you had a shower?' "Yes Why?" I replied. "Well, you haven't washed the back of your legs there is dirt on them".

Except it wasn't dirt, it was big black bruises about the size of two tennis balls on the back of each leg.

The Hyper-Speeds had probably caused Hyper-Bleeds and I must put this down to the shoes. I would never have guessed they could have had this sort of impact, but I believe they did. I did of course ignore all the warnings and guidelines so no fault on anyone but myself.

So these shoes looked and felt like the dogs' bollocks, but they turned out to be just bollocks for someone too heavy, too slow, and running too far. I have to own up to a self-inflicted injury here. Looking back, however, it would seem my 2015 choice of shoe was an inspirational move, and I would like to think I was a true pioneer in the emerging market for super shoes. Is it just a coincidence that Nike created the first 'super shoe' in 2016? (dream on).

By 2023 things have changed a lot from the good old days of dominance by Asics and Saucony. The famous Sub-2 attempt by Eliud Kipchoge in 2019 wearing Nike Zoom Vaporfly Elites created a market almost overnight as would be champions raced to find whatever time advantage they could. Athletics bodies also rushed to ban certain types of shoes for the elite runners while they worked out how much unfair advantage these shoes were giving. A review of recent podium winners for men and women in recent marathons shows there may now be a battle of the super shoes.

In 2019, Nike athletes took 31 of the 36 podium places in the six marathon majors. In 2023 the emergence of Adidas and the Adizero Adios Pro 3 took the top four places in the Boston Marathon men's race with the women's race winner running another brand called On.

It was estimated that more than half of the London Marathon 2023 field of 50,000 runners were running in 'super shoes'. The men's winner ran with the now 'old school' Nike Vaporfly, with second place running in the upgraded Alphafly. The third-place male and first-placed British male opted for Adidas. The first and second placed women ran Nike Alphafly with third running Adidas Adios Pro. No mention of Asics at this point!

As is the recurring theme of this book, I'm no expert, but a recent article in The Guardian quoted someone who is (Geoff Burns, biomechanics expert and sport physiologist for the US Olympic committee) with regard to the potential impact of the super shoes on a runners performance.

"Burns says that elite male athletes close to two hours are likely to receive up to three minutes of improvement, while for those in the 2:10-2:15 hour range it may be more like three to four minutes. The news for amateur runners in the 3:30 to four-hour range is even better. A pair of super shoes could cut their time by more than five minutes."

There has been a marked increase in the number of people running fast marathon times from 2013 to 2023 (see Chapter 26). Of the 230,000 runners that ran the Big Six marathons in 2013, only 3.5% went Sub-3. By 2013 this had almost doubled to 6.1%. Are we getting faster, fitter, lighter, stronger or is there something else at stake here.

If the shoe fits, wear it!

Having re-researched the Gel Hyper-Speeds and the new Vapor Fly's, the Hyper-Speeds are an ounce lighter than the Vapor Fly's and the descriptions of each are below.

Note to self: Stick with the Kyano's!

31.   Sub-3 Soundtrack

Tuning out from the crowd

For me a soundtrack is essential as you are going to need all the help you can get out there and for me it's about ballads and big hits and songs you can sing along to. The sound of the crowd (not meaning The Human League) is good for background noise except for anyone shouting, "You're nearly there" or "It's all downhill from here" at you. It's never all downhill and you are never almost there.

Remember, there will always be some mentally dark places during the race, and you will need to find something to help you hang on in there. The shoes you are wearing won't run themselves and the road you are running won't be downhill all the way with the wind behind you.

Back in the days before Spotify and iPhones the challenge was getting music into a digital format and uploading them to some sort of running device. For me the iPod was out, mostly because I worked for a PC company but also because there would be all that faffing around and having to have a subscription to iTunes, so it had to be something else.

I owned a vast record and CD collection, but you can't run with a CD Player strapped to your back and converting every CD to a digital file needed a proper converter and a hell of a a lot of time and patience.

Enter stage left, Mystic Chris, who was spending his life coming up with all sorts of new ideas and ways to go Sub-4 and who I had run Trailwalker with back in 2004.

Chris offered to convert my CD collection into a digital format for the price of him keeping a copy of the file. I had hundreds of CD's, and having vowed not to replace my whole vinyl collection with them, I had done exactly that. Chris was still keen, so I brought a suitcase full of CDs to work and handed them over.

After a few weeks Chris announced he had finished the first suitcase and I could now bring the second one. I think we ended up with four suitcases in all, and Chris painstakingly converted every single one of them into digital MP3 format. He proudly handed me over a hard drive about the size of a large cigarette case and I now had thousands of songs to choose from.

With content sorted, the next issue was the player. Every time I travelled abroad; I would scour the airport stores in search of the ultimate running device. I bought several over the years but the one I used most was a Samsung YP-F1. This was the size of your thumb with a built-in metal clasp like one of those old-fashioned money clips.

It lasted most of my running years but began to falter on me over time due to the amount of water being poured onto my head during races and the amount of ice being stuffed under my cap in the heat. I am pleased to report that it is still in my man drawer along with old phones, watches, torches, cameras, and cables that will never be used again but cannot be thrown away. I have managed to fire it back up for 'research' purposes and have included the Sub-3 song list still on it.

I'm not going to start going through the list and turn this into an episode of Desert Island Discs but there are a number of songs on here that have saved a Sub-3 attempt half-way through or near the end of a race when all else seemed lost. One song in particular needs a special mention for two reasons (1) Most marathons are run on a Sunday and (2) Endurance Life marathons, which are run on a Saturday, are always through old coastal towns and across wet sandy beaches. It also saved me near the end of the Tokyo marathon in 2013 and I played it over and over laying on the floor at the bag check after the race. Cue Morrisey.

Trudging slowly over wet sand
Back to the bench where your clothes were stolen
This is the coastal town
That they forgot to close down
Armageddon, come Armageddon
Come, Armageddon, come

Everyday is like Sunday
Everyday is silent and grey

Hide on the promenade, etch a postcard
"How I dearly wish I was not here"
In the seaside town
That they forgot to bomb
Come, come, come, nuclear bomb

Everyday is like Sunday
Everyday is silent and grey

Trudging back over pebbles and sand
And a strange dust lands on your hands

And on your face
On your face
On your face
On your face

Everyday is like Sunday
Win yourself a cheap tray
Share some greased tea with me
Everyday is silent and grey

2Pac - California love	Simple Minds - Don't You (Forget About Me)
Abba - I have a dream	Simple Minds - Mandela Day
Abba - Thank you for the music	SL2 - On a Ragga Tip
Abba - The name of the game	Snow Patrol - Chasing Cars
Billy Ocean - Love Really Hurts without you	Snow Patrol - Chocolate
Blondie - One way or another	Snow Patrol - Run
Blondie - Tide is High	Soft Cell - Say Hello Wave Goodbye
Bon Jovi - Always	Soft Cell - The Girl with the Patent Leather Face
Bon Jovi - Bed of Roses	Spandau Ballet - Through the barricades
Bon Jovi - Living on a Prayer	Spandau Ballet - True
Bon Jovi - Wanted Dead of Alive	Springsteen - Nebraska
Cold Play - The Scientist	Sting - Fields of Gold
Culture Club - The crying game	Stranglers - Nice 'N' Sleazy
Culture Club - Victims	Streophonics - Have a Nice Day
Depeche Mode - Photographic	Sylvester - You make me feel
Detroit Spinners - Working my way back to you	Take That - Patience
Double Trouble - Rebel MC - Street Tuff [Radio Mix]	Tavares - Don't take away the music
Earth Wind Fire - Boogie Wonderland	Tavares - Heaven Must be missing an angel
Elvis Costello & the Attractions - Two Little Hitlers	Tears for Fears - Mad World
Erasure - Ship of Fools	Tears for Fears - Shout
Fad Gadget - Back to nature	The Chimes - I Still Haven't Found What I'm Looking For
Gene Pitney/Soft Cell - Something's Gotten Hold of My Heart	The Clash - The Card Cheat
Green Day - Good Riddance (Time of Your Life)	The Clash - Train in Vain (Stand by Me)
Guns N Roses - Knocking on Heaven's Door	The Clash - What's My Name
Guns N' Roses - Sweet Child O' Mine	The Cure - Friday I'm in Love
JFK - Son of a Gun	The Jam - Ghosts
Kylie Minogue - Can't Get You Out Of My Head	The Jam - The Place I Love
L7 - Shitlist	The Jam - Butterfly Collector
Lady Gaga - Poker Face	The Lightning Seeds - You Showed Me
Madonna - Like a Prayer	The Rolling Stones - Beast of Burden
Madonna - Power of Goodbye	The Rolling Stones - Gimme Shelter
Manics - Design for life	The Rolling Stones - Just My Imagination
Meat Loaf - Two Out of Three Ain't Bad	The Rolling Stones - Wild Horses
Morrisey - Everyday is like Sunday	The Stranglers - Hanging Around
Oakenfold Feat. - Starry Eyed Surprise	The Tramps - Disco Inferno
Oasis - Don't Look Back in Anger	The Undertones - Teenage Kicks
OMD - Joan of Arc	The Vibrators - Baby Baby
OMD - Maid of Orleans	The Vibrators - Into the Future
Pet Shop Boys - What Have I Done to Deserve This	The Who - Baba O'Riley
Pulp - Common People	Thin Lizzy - Cowboy Song
Radiohead - Street Spirit [Fade Out]	U2 - I Still Haven't Found What I'm Looking For
Rod Stewart - The First Cut Is the Deepest	Visage - Fade to Grey
Roxette - It Must Have Been Love	Wham! - I'm Your Man

32. A Guinness World Record 2016 and Kona Guy

In the world of Ironman qualifying, for the annual world championships every October in Kona, Hawaii, is a similar, but not identical, quest for an amateur runner chasing a Sub-3 marathon. In 2003 when I completed my first Ironman, there were a dozen or so full Ironman races held worldwide and about 10,000 people had completed one.

Today, twenty years later, there are dozens of them around the world, in every country and sometimes two or more in countries big enough to hold them. Back in the day you would probably know someone who had run a marathon but no-one who had completed an Ironman. Today you probably know a dozen people who have completed both.

There is clearly a lot more to an Ironman than a marathon. Both have a registration day or two where you pick up your race number and your timing chip, then spend a lot of time and money buying things at the expo, that you don't need, and return to home or hotel to prepare for the race.

For a marathon it's probably a decent dinner and a good nights' sleep, up at dawn, get to the start, run for three hours, in the pub by lunchtime for beers and medals and to bore everyone to death with your race story. For an Ironman, there is a whole ton of stuff that needs doing before bedtime. Numerous numbers need to be stuck on bikes, helmets, and colour coded kit bags. Bikes must be tested and checked, and tyres pumped up to the right levels. Cycle gear needs to be put in a blue bag, running kit in a red bag, bikes and bags need to be taken to a racking area, also known as transition, at a designated time the day before the race. Bike and helmet checks are made against official wristbands before you must rack your bike in the right place and put each bag on the right pegs.

Anything you miss from a bag can mean race day disaster as it's not great to come out of the swim and realise you didn't put cycling shoes in the cycle bag. Timing chips are handed out upon exit from the racking at transition and you spend the rest of the day making sure you don't lose it, or on race morning forget it.

Nutrition in an Ironman is key to success. For a stand-alone marathon you can hold a Sub-3 marathon pace on water alone at scattered water stations, maybe a sip of energy drink here and there but you don't need more than that to do it.

For an average marathon you will burn around 2,500 calories, for a Sub-3 maybe 3,000+. For an Ironman its over 7,000 calories or closer to 10,000 for those elite runners going Sub-8 or Sub-9. Like marathons, there will be feeding stations on the bike and run whereas for the Ironman you can exchange drink bottles, take on gels, energy bars, and a variety of fruit and other stuff.

But for the most part you will rely on your main nutrition of choice which you can load on the bike the morning of the race and include in your race bags to use through each transition.

The elite and fast amateurs (like 'Good for Age') will typically stay calorie positive or neutral, their watches will beep to tell them to drink or eat so that they don't drop into a calorie deficit throughout the race. Nutrition being my weak point meant that of the fifteen Ironman races I completed, all were done with under one thousand calories and some as low as five hundred.

Each Ironman has several stated slots to be won for the upcoming World Championships the following October held in Kona Hawaii. Typically, there might be twenty or thirty slots or sometimes as many as two hundred. When the race entry deadlines have closed the number of slots is allocated by male and female and age-group categories. So, if you are a male 35-39 there maybe three slots available for Kona meaning you must finish in the top three of your age group.

The following day after each race, there is a Kona roll down where you must accept and pay for your slot there and then. If you came 2nd and either don't show or don't want it, then that slot would roll-down to the next person in the age group.

Qualifying for Kona is a step above a Sub-3 marathon in my opinion, though some of my Ironman mates would often disagree as most of them had never ran Sub-3 even though they were running 3:20-3:30 Ironman marathons. They also weren't that drawn to it as Ironman was their priority. We agreed at some point that a Sub-10 Ironman was probably equivalent to a Sub-3 marathon in terms of legendary status and a Sub-9, Sub-2:45 marathon was probably Elite status. Anything below that is pro level.

The debate and comparison are probably pointless but for the record my personal best was 11:03 and my typical time was closer to thirteen hours and longer.

So, a close Ironman friend of mine who shall be known as Kona Guy (who I met on my second ever Ironman in Florida) began his Ironman career like mine, running average times. We finished Florida in something over eleven hours each.

He, like me, caught the Ironman bug early on and made it an annual event to do at least one, sometimes two and even three Ironman races per year. Back in the day they were always abroad, and they often sold out within minutes of being opened for registration. So, they were costly not only because of all the kit to be bought but also the race fees and the travelling costs made me wonder why this sport was so popular.

As time went on, my times and performances gradually got worst as I got older and as the nutrition issue started to have an impact on my ability to even finish.

Kona Guy got faster as he got older, and it was soon apparent that he might be getting close to a Kona qualify. Like my quest for a Sub-3, could Kona Guy make Kona? He wasn't getting any younger and the sport was becoming more popular with more people doing it. In

March 2015 my worst nightmare came true. Kona Guy had qualified for Kona at South Africa Ironman in 4th place and in a time of Sub 10.30. Were the bragging rights about to shift?

Having made the Sub-3 cut in 2005, and many times since, I felt gave me bragging rights over him on what was otherwise simply finishing an Ironman which, quite frankly we've all done many times over. A Kona qualify turned the tables on that.

We only tended to meet up now and again at races or whenever he was in London and each time we met he would have his Kona race cap on and wear it throughout the day periodically asking if I owned one or not. I countered with the Sub-3 he had yet to achieve and for now there was an uneasy truce around what trumped what.

It was early 2016 and almost three years since I had run all six World Marathon Majors in 2013. I had managed to find a website that listed all of the 6 Star finishers and had double checked to see how many runners had done all six in 2013 given that was the first year it could have been done. I found about fifteen runners including myself. Looking through their times they were all four-hour type runners except another guy from Britain who had posted the odd Sub-3 but mostly three hours plus times.

I checked that all my times were quicker than his and more importantly what the New York times were, as whoever finished that first would be the first person in the world to run all six world majors in the same calendar year. The nightmare time I had posted of 3:00:01 was five minutes faster than the other Brit guy so that made me the first in the world to do it. I mentioned this at lunch, as you would, to a couple of work colleagues and one said, "Surely that's a Guinness record!", which got me thinking, surely a Guinness world record trumps a Kona qualify every day of the week.

I began to consider what this would mean. Kona Guy would turn up with his Kona cap on, whereas I would insist I only drink Guinness now (with my Guinness T-Shirt on) and on the hour every hour I would get my wife to phone me and let my newly found Roy Castle Record Breakers ring tone ring for a while before answering. I could even change my answer phone message to 'Hi, you're through to a Guinness world record holder, please leave a message after the tone'.

Every time Kona Guy phones me I can let it go to voicemail and every Xmas I can send him one of those Guinness world record albums signed by 'Yours Truly'. I wasn't letting this run away with me but as the delusional day went on, I was finding more ways in which to use this. All I needed was the bloody record!

On the 14th of March 2016 I applied for a Guinness World Record under the title: 'Fastest aggregate time to complete every annual World Marathon Majors Marathon'. You couldn't invent a title you had to select one and this was the nearest one. There were lots of rules and guidance and the need to upload evidence, but this looks good.

I wasted no time contacting Kona Guy to seek his thoughts and to start planning what his life would soon be like. He listened to my evidence and rationale and reluctantly he felt it was credible and yes, he had watched Record Breakers as a kid and no he didn't drink Guinness and he would text me in future rather than phone.

I uploaded all the evidence, explained that this could only be done in 2013 given Tokyo's new status, I shared all the details of all the runners who had run Tokyo that year as well as the other five majors. I explained the rationale and waited for a response.

A month or so later, following, a chase up, I received the reply that it had been rejected as it wasn't about being the first but the fastest. I asked why Roger Bannister was still on their website given he was the first to run a Sub-4-minute mile but was no longer the fastest. I also pointed out that I was indeed the fastest to do all six in 2013 based on my aggregate time being the fastest, and the fact I had been the fastest finisher in all six individually.

They noted my Roger Bannister observation and doubled down on the fastest criteria meaning it could be in any year. I battled away with them for a while before eventually giving up on the discussion as they simply wouldn't see it. Which is a bit of a let-down, given the ridiculous number of runners you now see at the London Marathon with "Official Guinness World Record Attempt" banners pinned on them.

These attempts can range from "Fastest Tomato" or "Fastest in a Mankini" or "Fastest Vicar". All you have do is think of a new category and the be fastest (or most probably the first and only).

I appreciate you may see this as churlish, and I do understand the point about being the fastest vs the first. I do get it. But I was the fastest to run all six in the same year in 2013 at least and there were 71 official Guinness World Record attempts at the London marathon in 2023 including the following which I struggle to see as being of equal calibre. Maybe I am being picky!

Fastest marathon dressed in pyjamas (male)
Fastest marathon dressed as a fisher
Fastest marathon dressed as a postal worker (male)
Fastest marathon dressed as a knight (male)
Fastest marathon wearing clogs (male)
Fastest marathon dressed as a star (male)
Fastest marathon in a Kung Fu uniform
Fastest marathon dressed as a lifeguard (male)
Fastest marathon dressed as reptile (female)
Fastest marathon dressed as a key (male)
Fastest marathon dressed as a road vehicle (male)
Fastest marathon dressed as a monarch (male)
Fastest marathon by a mascot (male)
Fastest marathon dressed as a milk deliverer (male)
Fastest marathon dressed as an insect (male)
Fastest marathon dressed as a scientist (male)
Fastest marathon dressed in pyjamas (female)
Fastest marathon dressed as a postal worker (male)
Fastest marathon dressed as a mammal (male)
Fastest marathon dressed as a gingerbread person
Fastest marathon in highland dress (male)

Fastest marathon dressed as a mammal (female)
Fastest marathon in a toga (male)
Fastest marathon dressed as a book (male)
Fastest marathon dressed as a body part (female)
Fastest marathon dressed in pyjamas (female)
Fastest marathon dressed as a scientist (male)
Fastest marathon dressed as a can (male)
Fastest marathon dressed as a lumberjack (male)
Fastest marathon dressed as a book (male)
Fastest marathon dressed in a safari suit (male)
Fastest marathon dressed as a lumberjack (male)
Fastest marathon dressed as a crustacean (female)
Most underpants worn during a marathon (female)
Fastest marathon dressed as a food jar / tub (male)
Fastest marathon dressed as a pirate (female)
Fastest marathon dressed as a glass (male)
Fastest marathon dressed as a glass (female)
Fastest marathon dressed as a boxer
Fastest marathon dressed as a vegetable (female)
Fastest marathon in a four-person costume
Fastest marathon in a two-person costume
Fastest marathon dressed as a body part (male)
Fastest marathon in a three-person costume
Fastest marathon dressed as a golfer (male)
Fastest marathon carrying golf clubs (male)

I have also noticed that the "Most Underpants worn during a marathon" record didn't seem to have the fastest element to it so I may have to appeal this ruling against me at some point although I wasn't wearing any underpants during my races in 2013.

I have included this list to serve as a point of comparison between my noteworthy claim for a record and these somewhat less serious categories. I hope this hasn't given you any similar unworthy ideas to make the record books.

I have since cancelled my subscription to The Guinness World Record Book club, and I no longer drink Guinness as a protest. I am reliably informed that their profits are down significantly since taking these actions.

As for Kona Guy, he seems to be getting faster by age not slower. At the time of writing this, Kona Guy had qualified for Kona every time in his last four races and was 1st and 3rd age group finisher in his last two races with his Ironman PB standing at 9:42 which to some extent supports the Sub-10 is a Sub-3 debate we had many years ago.

From: noreply@guinnessworldrecords.com
Date: 14 March 2016 at 13:04:37 GMT
Subject: Guinness World Records Application
Accepted
Application Reference: 160130181041ftra

Hello Andrew

We are pleased to inform you that your application has been accepted under the following title: Fastest aggregate time to complete every annual World Marathon Majors marathon.

When you visit your online Application Summary using the link below, you will be able to view both the details of the current record to beat (or minimum requirement for an open record title) and the Record Guidelines for this record title.

The Record Guidelines detail the rules which must be followed during your attempt for this Guinness World Records title. Each point of the Guidelines must be followed by anyone attempting this record.

If you do not follow the Record Guidelines or do not provide all the evidence we request, your application may be rejected.

You need to upload all the documents listed in the Evidence checklist on the Application Summary.

Good luck with your record attempt and we look forward to receiving your evidence.

Kind regards

Records Management Team

Guinness World Records

33. Barcelona Marathon 2016
Sub-3 Vs Post-2

So, a common debate amongst friends when announcing what time you did, would require the key first number out of your mouth being '2' with the rest not being that relevant as that designated a Sub-3.

For the Barcelona Marathon of 2016 I stayed in a hotel a few minutes' walk from the start/finish line so a perfect location for the start, and an easy hobble back for a shower afterwards with time to get back to the finish to watch my niece who was also running. I was aware of a group of African runners also staying at the hotel, so I wondered who they were as I'm not someone who can name or recognise any of the top world marathon runners.

After a dismal race, and a blow-up on time closer to my Sub-4 days, I found myself in the lift going up to the room with one of the elite African runners. He had a sash on saying first place and was carrying a large trophy so clearly this was fast company. I acknowledged him in the lift, marvelled at his achievement, and ambled off for a shower.

On the way back down, I was joined in the lift by three other elite African runners along with their friends all dressed up and ready to go out and celebrate their race. I simply had to ask the question. "What time did you do?" I was clearly expecting them to say "2" and something.

The main guy I was talking to clearly didn't understand what I was saying so I said it again and this time pointed at my watch. Not sure why I thought that would help him but by now his friends were also listening. One of them appeared to translate to him and he said in broken English "10.08". That's all he said. I guess that's all he needed to say.

For him "2" is not the issue as that's a done deal, for him it's down to how many minutes over "2" that counts. I let out a gasp of appreciation and asked the same thing of his two colleagues. One said "10.23" the other said "11.19". I was in the lift with three sporting heroes who I could neither name nor identify but for whom any discussion or bragging rights around a Sub-3 would be completely lost on them.

I still have the photos of them, and their friends taken as we got out of the lift. I guess Sub-3 is still something for us mortals as it's an hours issue whereas for the immortals like them it's a minutes thing!

For the record these were three Kenyan athletes who finished 2nd, 3rd and 4th and their names were Albert Korir, Jafred Kipchumba and Eliud Taurus. The winner in the lift on the way up was Dino Safir from Ethiopia who probably would have said "9.31" had I asked him the same question.

34. London Marathon 2017
The End of Something!

Having begun this quest back in 1990 or even as far back as 1981, when I was first rejected from competing based on a timed postmark, this had become a part of my sporting life for more than twenty-five years. A backdrop challenge supporting more important sports such as football, rugby, and triathlon it was a constant companion and a periodic chance to do something special. If Sub-3 was the constant goal, then at what stage or time would it be time to call it a day?

When would the simple act of running a marathon no longer be the point? Like the laddish bet of 1990 there had to be a reverse position of when to quit and sometime during the 10-year golden era of running one or more Sub-3's every year I announced to myself that the time to quit was a post-4.

Although it was becoming clear that a Sub-3 and the S3XX tattoo were both slipping from sight, the spectre of a post-4 was surely years away. My pace and performance was slipping and though this was still eighteen months before I would receive a CLL cancer diagnosis, a condition I could have been suffering from since well before 2017, there had to be a line in the sand and the line had been drawn.

Deep down I was expecting to lose the coveted Good for Age guarantee at some point but having dipped inside the time in 2016 which provided a further two years of entries the target time of 3:20 had to be hit to hold that position going forward.

I felt fine the day of the race and went through the well-trodden path of leaving the house, getting the district line to Embankment, walking up to Charing Cross, boarding the train to Blackheath, ambling to the start, using the loo at the same coffee shop off the beaten track from the masses of other runners, into the Good for Age pen, queue for the loo again, bag drop, headphones, bin liner, foot right on the start line, away we go.

There were no familiar faces at the start line like in previous year's. Runners who you would suddenly remember as you were running alongside them wearing the same vest or with the same old headband seemed absent. Ironman races were becoming fewer and farther between and I was getting a few DNF's and questioning why I was bothering and what was the point anymore.

But there was still the hanging thought of twenty Sub-3's even though it had been three years now since the last Sub-3 finish.

I don't remember much about the race. I crossed halfway well outside 1:30 but there was still hope of a Sub-3:20 to make the qualifying time as I had marginally done the year before.

By the time I made it to the start of the Embankment section, any hope of a qualifying time was well and truly gone, and other runners were passing me in droves as my pace was clearly declining fast. As we made the turn

205

at Big Ben, I was beginning to realise that a Sub-4 was now in doubt, or maybe I was reading it wrong, it didn't seem to matter either way at the time. I assumed it was going to be a bad three hour something, finish.

As I finally crossed the line with other runners racing to finish and checking their watches, I simply had to check the clock as I had started with my foot on the start line, so the watch time is the clock time unlike those around me who were probably trying to dip under 3:30 or something.

If it had been 3:59:59 it would have been a blessing and a reason to go again, but it was 4:00:20 and it was the end of something.

Twenty-one seconds spelled the end of twenty-five years of doing this.

Maybe it was a blessing as this would be the last marathon I would ever run, and the quest was finally over.

I walked back along to the bag truck and joined the masses and carried on through to the arches at the end of the Mall and disappeared down to the tube to get the ride back to West London and that was that.

The end of something.

35. Cancer, Sepsis, and the loss of pace and power.

There was a noticeable loss to my pace and power based on my deteriorating Ironman times and my increasing tendency to DNF after the bike or early into the run. The indignity of going over four hours at the London Marathon the previous year was a clear sign of age catching up with me and any chance of a S3XX tattoo was all but gone. Surely there was no way back from a four-hour-plus finish? Taking off 15-20 minutes maybe, taking an hour off, no way.

I was doing less training and running fewer races from the crazy times of 2011-13 where I was running upwards of twelve marathons a year mixed with Endurance Life, marathon majors and Ironman marathons. Ironman was giving way to challenges like the Long Course Weekend in Wales which included The Wales Marathon.

This was a more relaxed 'Ironman' with the individual disciplines spread over 3 days, so swim – go to pub, cycle – go to pub, run – go to pub or go home. But even for this the marathon leg was proving tougher and I could feel my pace and power draining away from what was probably just old age and not training as much and enjoying a few glasses of wine every night.

In November 2018 I decided to clear out an old shed in the garden and my brother Glenn helped take it down to ship it out ready for a new replacement. I worked my way through the tins of paint, the old gardening tools and the spider's webs and eggs to clear it out ready for the demolition in the next day or two.

Later that day I was aware of some sort of bite on the top of head and was picking away at it. My wife immediately blamed it on a false widow spider as she was, and is, convinced that they are everywhere and that sooner or later they might bite the dog and it could die and that my flesh would soon begin to deteriorate, and I could lose a limb if I didn't get it treated. I couldn't see a spider bringing down a life-long athlete, so I brushed it off as an old wives' tale.

A day or so later I felt what I thought was a big spot, or boil, just behind my ear and was attempting to lance it with a needle when my wife caught up with proceedings and announced the spot was my lymph nodes so lancing them with a needle wasn't textbook treatment. She went on to explain that lymph nodes are there to fight infection and that clearly, she was right about the spider and that I should go to the doctor's pronto the following day. I checked in for an appointment and they took some blood for testing and sent me on my way.

A few days later the doctor called asking me to come back in as they needed to take another blood test as the results had come back and my white blood cell count was too high, so they needed to test again to make sure all was back to normal. Another needle in the arm later and a list of ten questions to answer, all of which were 'no', and off I went. A few days later the doctor called again and said the white cell count was higher not lower than the previous test and she asked the same ten questions again which were still 'No'. She only seemed mildly concerned but instructed me to call back if my temperature went up.

A few nights later I had a mild sweat, and my wife stuck a thermometer gauge in my ear and said I should call the doctor later that morning to explain the temperature change. I was feeling fine and better, so I forgot to phone until about lunchtime when I was driving around the local area doing some shopping. The doctor came on the phone; I said my temperature had been 38.9 or whatever my wife had written down for me, and she said, "You need to go to A&E immediately, I will inform them you are coming but go there now".

It was a Thursday lunchtime, and this seemed a bit dramatic for what began as a pussy-spot, but it seemed serious so off I went. Having checked in to A&E and explained what the doctor had told me I sat in reception waiting and wondering what the fuss was all about.

I was called quickly and taken through the check in routine before being taken down a ward and placed on a bed. The A&E doctor arrived and asked me the similar ten questions as the GP doctor had been asking. "Are you in Pain?" "Have you lost weight?" "Feeling tired?" "Are your glands up?" "Is your temperature up?" "Discomfort in your stomach?" "Fatigue?" "Short of breath?" "Regular infections?" and I answered 'No' to all of them.

Blood samples were taken, temperature checks and various other things, before the next thing I know they are setting up a drip and putting me on bottle one of two. My worried wife turned up an hour or so later asking what's wrong and whether she should get stuff in case they keep me in. I said, no chance, I feel fine and once the drip is all done and a few tests then I should be out.

The doctor re-appeared and disclosed what the problem might be. Sepsis. At this point I had no idea what sepsis was, and my wife wasn't that sure either but the doctor stated that I would need to be held in over-night, under observation, and would be moved to a ward once the drips were done. All seemed odd and once the doctor had gone, we started Googling 'sepsis' to get the low down.

A few weeks after all of this I was at a dinner party with some friends, and I was telling someone what had happened and that they initially thought I had sepsis, and I was making light of it all.

The person I was talking to went very quiet and very serious and told me that a young relative of his, who had initially contracted a dental infection and the delay in diagnosing sepsis meant she had lost her life within twenty-four hours of being admitted as the hospital frantically fought to stop the spread.

Sepsis is a life-threatening blood poisoning disorder and has a 40% mortality rate. More people die from sepsis than cancer and from what I can tell it starts with people (like me) taking symptoms lightly and hospitals or doctors not diagnosing it soon enough.

Sepsis can kill you within twelve hours and looking back I can see why the doctor said go to straight to A&E and why the hospital got me onto a drip quickly.

I was never diagnosed with sepsis. I was blood tested five or six more times on Thursday and throughout Friday as each new doctor on shift came to see me, they asked me the same ten questions again and wanted another sample to test for something else.

Eventually I insisted on being discharged that Friday evening as my arm was full of holes and I hadn't got any more blood to give. Plus, I don't like needles. I promised to come straight back if there were any symptoms and we returned on Sunday a bit concerned when they took more blood tests and tested for a variety of other things including AIDS.

Eventually they sent me to the Haematology unit at Hammersmith Hospital and I was finally diagnosed as having CLL or Chronic Lymphatic Leukaemia which is a blood cancer involving a high white cell blood count. They couldn't say when I had contracted this condition. It could have been months ago or more likely years ago.

It is very common for middle to older age people to have CLL but not find out until they have a random blood test. Could this have been caused by the damaged blood cells in 2015 and the year of running in the wrong shoes? Could the sheer volume of running and training and a high stress job all combined have brought it on? No-one knows and I don't spend time thinking about it.

A friend of my wife's husband also has it, or had it, but much worse than me. He was unable to walk a flight of stairs without falling short of breath and had started treatment some time earlier. My condition was, and still is, very mild.

I have a check-up every six months and although my white cell count is always too high it is compensated by the other aspects of my blood condition. If nothing else, it may explain, or give me the perfect excuse, to blame my more recent drop of pace, power, and performance on CLL rather than my age and my reduced level of training.

I have stopped running almost completely since 2019/2020. I don't miss it. Having spent years and years running day in day out in all weathers and all temperatures and on holidays, during work events, on Xmas Eve, Xmas Day, and Boxing Day, on birthdays, weddings, funerals, and christenings, in ice, snow, sand, mud, through rivers, forests, up and down mountains, through major cities, towns and village marathons and everywhere you can think of.

I have run the University Boat Race course along the river from Hammersmith to Kew, up to Putney and back to Hammersmith probably more than 2,000 times since I moved there in 1990 and still live there thirty years later.

I have run almost 100 competitive marathons and probably a distance of two marathons a week every week to train for it. I think I have done enough running and whoever Forrest Gump is then I have run whatever he ran 100 times over. CLL may be a way of someone somewhere telling me to slow down and do something else.

For the last few years, I have been struggling along with Ironman 70.3 races timed to coincide with my son doing the full distance. I get through the swim and bike and walk the run for the most part and I don't care if I am last to finish. Running is no longer a holy grail.

I did a bit of research for this as I feel it is something that should be taken seriously and understood. I read a blog from someone in March 2019, and he wrote,

"Let's go back to the beginning for a moment: like most people, my CLL was only discovered by accident during a routine blood test with a GP following the flu", sounds familiar, but he continued with "unlike the average age population patient population with this, I was only 39 years old".

So, it can happen much earlier than mid to old age and is typically only diagnosed by accident which may feel comforting but can be scary for friends and family when they discover you have it. CLL is a potentially life-threatening condition but thank God it wasn't sepsis.

I don't want to alarm people about sepsis but if I had had it when they admitted me to A&E then maybe this memoir wouldn't have been written.

Maybe if you are struggling to find something to run for then run for a charity that supports research into it. Here are some things to consider.

- Someone in the United States is diagnosed with sepsis every 20 seconds.
- The risk of dying from sepsis increases by as much as 8% for every hour of delayed treatment.
- On average, approximately 30% of patients diagnosed with severe sepsis do not survive.

I have included a page of something I found on the internet regarding the stages of sepsis. As I said, despite two days of tests at the hospital, they were not able to pin down what was wrong. This disease or condition is more common than you think, and it can go from bad to very worse in a matter of hours so don't take any chances for yourself of anyone else who may have it.

Stage One: Sepsis
Sepsis can be hard to identify in its early stages, common symptoms that show evidence of it during its first stage include:

- A high fever above (38°C) or low temperature below (36°C)
- A heart rate above 90 beats per minute
- A bacterial, fungal, or viral infection confirmed with positive blood culture results
- Rapid breathing rate higher than 20 Breaths per minute

The sooner you receive medical care, the higher your chances for survival. If caught before it affects vital organs, it's possible to treat the infection with antibiotic therapy. Most people who have sepsis detected at this stage make a full recovery.

Stage Two: Severe Sepsis

The second stage of sepsis, severe sepsis, is diagnosed when life-threatening organ dysfunction happens characterized by symptoms or vital signs, including:

- Abnormal heartbeat or poor cardiac output
- Decreased urine output
- Sudden changes in mental state
- Difficulty breathing or acute respiratory distress syndrome
- Abnormal pain
- Chills due to reduced body temperature
- Extreme weakness
- Unconsciousness and confusion

Stage Three: Septic Shock

Patients transitioning to stage 3 are said to be in septic shock, the most dangerous phase of sepsis. The symptoms of septic shock are like those in stage two, including perfusion abnormalities (e.g., elevated lactate levels). This stage has the highest chance of mortality, with estimates ranging between 30% and 50%.

36. The Power of 10

Many years ago, I stumbled across a website called Power of 10 which is run by British Athletics. The chances are you are already on it if you have run a major marathon and you are most probably on it if you have run a minor marathon.

I don't know how they choose what races to include on it, but you can also submit a result with evidence and eventually they will include it once verified. It has all your results including half marathons, ultra's, 10K's, weird distances, the lot. You should check it out if you have run any races recently.

There is an additional sister site called Run Britain and when you log in to that you get all sorts of graphs and rankings and statistics about where you rank by category of sex, age, distance and so on. In 2013 it shows my ranking as top 2.1% based on a 2:56 Tokyo finish and at 1.9% in 2011 based on 2:57 Dublin. In 2017 and the end of something year it shows me at 34.7% with a London time of 4:00:23. It's a very cool site and I don't think its existence is widely known.

I searched for James Cracknell, and it shows he missed a Sub-3 by just 10 seconds in London 2006 before he made it by just by 48 seconds in 2008 and then went sub 2:45 in 2017 so major respect and credit for an Elite finish of 2:45. He was still Sub-3ing in 2021 and from what I can see he has Sub-3'd around six times throughout his new running career.

My Power of 10

I'm not sure what the main point of this book was and why anyone should care, and, in some ways, I still feel that way. I was never a runner by any stretch of the imagination and as I said at the start I began life as a footballer, changed to rugby, then to triathlon. I simply ran to keep fit for another sport and marathons were a good way to test yourself in between games or races.

In 2005 at the age of forty-four I finally managed to go Sub-3 in Dublin after fifteen years of trying and it was more satisfying than any football or rugby trophy winning moment or even an Ironman finish.

I had expected to call it a day after the emotion of finally doing it once, as there were more important things to focus on, but I seemed to be getting faster with age and it took on a whole life of its own.

I have lost count of the number of marathons I have run but I think its two or three shy of one hundred. The only record worth keeping though seemed to be those that were done in Sub-3 and those in really special places around the world like The Great Wall in China.

If I had a personal 'Power of 10' then it would have to be the fact that I managed to Sub-3 every year for ten consecutive years between 2005 and 2014.

Sadly the quest for a S3XX tattoo to signify twenty Sub-3's didn't happen. I came up short with just seventeen.

Perhaps had the new 'super shoes' (See Chapter 30) with a potential four or five-minute advantage been around in those days then who knows maybe twenty-five Sub-3's would have been on the cards.

Looking back on it now, the time and sacrifice to maintain that level of pace and fitness at that age and for that long is something I am very proud of.

The friends I have met and raced with along the way and the support from family and work colleagues for the past three decades has been life changing.

It's difficult to put it into more meaningful words so I won't bother trying as it will turn out cheesy and naff. Maybe the PB's below speak for themselves. It was whatever it was.

2005	Dublin	02:58:48	2010	Dublin	02:52:57
2006	London	02:53:00	2011	Dublin	02:57:39
2007	London	02:51:14	2012	Dublin	02:58:58
2008	London	02:46:30	2013	Tokyo	02:56:41
2009	London	02:46:59	2014	London	02:57:36

37.   My Top 10 tips

I am conscious that this book has not provided specific tips on how to run a Sub-3 marathon as to be honest I don't think I have much to offer in this space given it took me so long to do it. You probably want quicker results than that.

Going Sub-3 is not about being a 'good runner'. Running is simply the act of walking faster. Put one foot in front of the other without falling over. There is no recognised running style needed to run a fast marathon except maybe to run forwards vs running up and down.

I would, however, offer one overall thing to think about as well as a quick list of tips on the final page. Don't set one goal, set three or four and rank them if you can. This can increase over time if you are starting out with one goal but looking back I ended up with three goals that had to be hit every year from about 2011 onwards.

These goals were in priority rank order as follows

1) Complete an Ironman (finish critical)
2) Run a Sub-3 Marathon (time critical)
3) Podium Endurance Life (position critical)

These were three very different goals, each of which came with a different problem.

Ironman racing for me was more about a finish than a time as my inability to get fuel and nutrition down during the race meant it was pointless expecting a decent time, or finishing before the hours of darkness, and certainly not a Kona qualify chance.

I think I have covered the Sub-3 issue.

Endurance Life races are tough in themselves whether taking on the Marathon or Ultra distance. It's completely different to flat road racing and each course is wildly different so a place finish becomes more important than a time finish and given there being less than two-hundred people running then, based on percentages, a podium finish was always possible unless a group of serious fell runners turned up and blew everyone off.

Today in 2023, I am over sixty, back to 83kg and cycling just an hour every evening in the garage watching the TV. I don't really miss those running days, I feel exhausted just thinking about them. I am the proud owner of an arthritic hip and I suspect the CLL isn't helping any. I am probably ready for the knacker's yard.

I have completed three half-ironman (70.3) races in the past year (2022) but sadly not all within the 8-hour cut-off time due to my walking performances on the running leg. I am simply out there on the course to support my son and other friends who are normally doing the full distance on the same day or weekend.

My niece recently completed her first triathlon at the age of eleven and my son his fourth Ironman in Italy. I have finally taken up golf to keep up with my two sons who tell me they have both "shot a birdie". It sounds more relaxing.

There are plenty of guides and guidance on how to be good at running written and explained by people more informed and experienced than me. They all have their part to play and their advice to follow. But if you were expecting a few tips from me at least, then here are a few things you might consider.

1) Vary what you do, swimming, cycling, strength training, trail marathons, triathlons.
2) Build your sport around your life not your life around your sport.
3) Run lots of half marathons during normal training runs. At least one a week.
4) Enter at least five marathons per year. Don't rely on getting into the world majors.
5) Set a 1:25 half marathon target and achieve that first then hold Sub 1:30 training runs.
6) Lose some weight, even if it's just a few pounds or kilos. We are all too heavy.
7) Don't obsess with the race clock, know your Sub-3 pace by heart.
8) Sort out your inspirational play list no matter how embarrassing and zone out of everything else.
9) Get OK with nutrition, don't overdo it. It's a three-hour race not a weeklong camping expedition.
10) Always tell your friends you are going Sub-3 no matter how ridiculous it may sound or feel.

Best of luck. You can do this. And remember,

A road is for running no matter how far or fast you run it.

Special thanks and references

Peter G.J.M Janssen - Training Lactate Pulse-Rate
The Serpentine Triathlon and Running Club
Endurance Life @endurancelife.com
The Power of 10 @thepowerof10.info
Mystic Chris and Modest Martin
Sauce and Wildman
Elmbridge Guy
The Jonesy's, Kona Guy, Rhino Guy, and families
Guinness World Records @guinnessworldrecords.com
World Marathon Majors @worldmarathonmajors.com
The Toshiba Corporation
Runners World @forums.runnersworld.co.uk
Mr Mouse Farm and Tough Guy Alumni
Boston Strong
Dublin, Buswells, Run4Janice team and family.
Extreme Running Ltd and Map Books generally
The Guardian - Super Shoes
Geoff Burns – US Olympic committee
Samsung MP3 players
Ironman distance racing
Morrisey #everydayislikesunday
Masseurs everywhere
Daniel Abrahams @Linked-In
Book Printing UK @bookprintinguk.com
Sally

Printed in Great Britain
by Amazon